THE NURSING OF THE
DYING PA

Other Books from Beaconsfield Publishers

Behavioural Science in Medicine
Helen Winefield, PhD & Marilyn Peay, PhD, 1980

Caring at Home for a Dying and Disabled Person
Professor Eric Wilkes, FRCP, in preparation

The First Words Language Programme
Bill Gillham, BA, DipPsych, 1979

Homoeopathic Prescribing
Dr Noel Pratt, 1980

Homoeopathy in Practice
Dr Douglas Borland, ed. Dr Kathleen Priestman, 1982

Introduction to Homoeopathic Medicine
Dr Hamish Boyd, FRCP, 1981

The Medical Report and Testimony
Gerald Pearce, FRCS, 1979

Stoma Care
ed. Brigid Breckman, SRN, RSCN, JBCNS (Stoma Care), 1981

Surgery and Your Heart
Donald Ross, FRCS & Barbara Hyams, MA, 1982

Take Care of Your Elderly Relative
Dr Muir Gray, MD & Heather McKenzie, LLB, 1980

The Nursing Care of the Dying Patient

'In the Midst of Life'

Alison Charles-Edwards
SRN, HV, JBCNS (Terminal Care)

BEACONSFIELD PUBLISHERS LTD
Beaconsfield, Bucks, England

British Library Cataloguing in Publication Data

Charles-Edwards, Alison
The nursing care of the dying patient.
1. Terminal care
I. Title
362.1'96029   R726.8

ISBN 0-906584-08-6

Phototypeset by Prima Graphics, Camberley, Surrey, in 9 and 10 point Times.
Printed in Great Britain at the University Press, Oxford

*Dedicated to my father,
the late Owen Parry*

Preface

Although a great deal of literature has been published recently concerning the care of the dying, much of this has been written from a psychological, sociological or spiritual vantage point. Consequently, there still appeared to be a need for a book covering the whole kaleidoscope of terminal care, and this is the gap I have attempted to fill. It seemed essential to provide the fundamental information about the control of symptoms, the physical aspects of nursing and the many practical matters, such as financial aid and what to do after someone has died, as well as describing the psychosocial response. The complete range of needs must be viewed together if patients and their relatives are to be treated as 'whole people' and cared for effectively.

When writing this book, I was doing so with nurses very much in the forefront of my mind, whether they were working in the community, in a hospital or in a hospice. However, a great deal of what I have written may be of equal value to other health care workers or, indeed, to the lay public, especially those involved in caring for a dying person.

On several occasions I have been critical of prevailing attitudes towards the dying and the standard of care which they receive. However, I have tried to offset each criticism with constructive suggestions for an alternative approach, and I am fully aware that many patients, both in their own homes and in hospital wards, receive the highest standard of care attainable.

I must acknowledge the fact that I have made no attempt to describe the care of terminally ill children. This is not because I feel it to be of any lesser importance, but rather because my own experience is too limited, and because specialist work in this field is still in an embryonic stage. The world's first two children's hospices are already coming into operation in Oxford and New York, so it should not be long now before we have a sound body of information about symptom control in children to add to the present literature on their psychosocial needs. Nevertheless, many of the general principles of caring for the dying apply equally to both children and adults, so paediatric nurses may well find the book to be of some value.

There were many occasions in the course of writing this text where the use of a singular, third person pronoun was called for. To avoid the clumsiness of 'he or she' on each occasion, I have quite arbitrarily referred to all nurses as 'she', all doctors as 'he', and all patients as 'he', except in the case of specifically female patients. I would, therefore, like to acknowledge the existence and value of my male nursing and female medical colleagues, and trust that they will not find this too irksome.

Similarly, when referring to the people most closely involved with a patient, I have frequently classified them as 'family' or 'relatives' for the sake of clarity and simplicity. However, many patients have friendships which are more important to them than their family relationships, so whenever the family is mentioned, please interpret it as 'those who are closest to the patient'.

One final explanation of the semantics in this book is needed to clarify the use of the word 'community'. I have used it in the dubious manner conventional amongst health care professionals, meaning anything outside hospital. Ideally, hospitals should be an integral part of the community in which they are situated, so it is to be hoped that this use will eventually fade and be replaced by something less divisive.

In Chapters 6 and 7, which are concerned with the management of pain and other common symptoms, a large number of drugs are mentioned. However, this collection does not purport to be a comprehensive list of all the possible drug-therapies available – it simply offers a selection of those which I have seen prescribed with good effect, with their normal dose range. It is to be anticipated that some of the drugs mentioned will be superseded within the lifetime of this book. The majority of drugs have certain contra-indications and some will interact unfavourably with other drugs. In addition, dosage varies widely from patient to patient. It must be stressed, therefore, that no one other than the physician, who has a complete picture of his patient's medical condition, is in a position to decide which drug and what dose is the safest and best choice.

In the same two chapters, the following abbreviations are used:

ml	millilitre	tabs	tablets
mg	milligram	o.d.	daily
g	gram	b.d.	twice daily
i.u.	international unit	t.d.s.	three times daily
i.m.	intramuscular	q.d.s.	four times daily
i.v.	intravenous	mane	in the morning
s.c.	subcutaneous	nocte	at night
p.o.	orally	stat	immediately
p.r.	rectally	p.r.n.	as required
p.v.	vaginally		

All proprietary names are written with an initial capital letter, whilst non-proprietary (generic) names are written with small letters.

Although I have nursed dying patients on general hospital wards and in their own homes, I have also had the privilege of working in three different hospices, and much of the information I am attempting to pass on and many of the experiences I am sharing were obtained in one or other of these units. If, as a result of reading this book, insight into the feelings and reactions of those approaching death and the competence and confidence to care for them effectively is increased just a little, I shall feel that I have begun to repay my debt to all the patients, relatives and colleagues who have given me so much.

I have both needed and received a great deal of advice and encouragement in order to write this book and I would like to express my gratitude to those who have helped me. I am particularly grateful to Kay Wells, organiser of the Social Care of the Gravely Ill at Home Project, Kent; Richard Hillier, consultant physician to Countess Mountbatten House, Southampton; Pat Young, editor of *Geriatric Medicine*; Margaret Pollock and John Caley of the Joint Board of Clinical Nursing Studies; Don Gillyett, pharmacist, John Radcliffe Hospital, Oxford; Donald Richards, hospital practitioner, Sir Michael Sobell House, Oxford; Marjory Cockburn, matron, St Luke's Nursing Home, Sheffield; Muir Gray, community physician, Oxford; Jacqueline Flindall, district nursing officer, Oxford; Elizabeth Janes, clinical nurse specialist in nutrition, Royal Marsden Hospital; Jim Crow, marketing consultant—clinical nutrition; Tom Snee, Nursing Officer, DHSS, London; Nora Snee, community liaison nurse, Royal Marsden Hospital; and Geoff Parkinson, a friend who works in the publishing business, all of whom ploughed their way through earlier or later drafts and showered me with constructive criticism and encouragement.

I should also like to take this opportunity to thank four of my former colleagues to whom this book and I owe a great deal; Eileen Mann, the first matron of St Luke's Nursing Home, Sheffield, and Robert Twycross, consultant physician to Sir Michael Sobell House, Oxford, for all that they taught me; Joan Steel, sometime ward sister of St Christopher's Hospice, London, and Viv Pritchard, nursing officer of Sir Michael Sobell House, Oxford, whose standards of nursing inspired me.

I am deeply indebted to John Churchill, my publisher, for his patience and for having such confidence in me. I would also like to thank Brenda Marshall for her thorough copy-editing of the final manuscript.

And finally I would like to thank my family, without whose help and support I could not have written this book, but especially my husband, David, who gave me the courage to keep writing, and Heather, my sister, who typed all four drafts and coped with my life-long problem of spelling.

                                                          A.C.-E.

Contents

Chapter 1

The Death Taboo

To be close to someone who is dying is to look death full in the face. Most people living in the Western hemisphere at the present time are particularly adept at avoiding such direct confrontation; hence the all-too-frequent alienation and isolation of those who are soon to die. Before embarking upon the care of a dying person, it is essential to explore one's own understanding of, and feelings about, death. Without this preparation, the barrier to any real depth of communication may be quite impenetrable.

Anyone encountering death will inevitably be led to some acknowledgement of their own mortality and, subsequently, to the arousal of the survival instinct. Fear of one's own demise and death can be so overwhelming that it is not possible to perceive the needs of the dying person or to share in his feelings. This may seem unlikely and hard to accept, since the fears are usually buried far below the level of conscious recognition; but it could hardly be demonstrated more clearly than it was by the patient who said, 'I never knew fear until I saw it in the eyes of those caring for me'.

Unfamiliarity with death has now become the norm. Many people reaching middle age have never encountered it, unless they happen to work with the sick or have seen active military service. The incidence of premature deaths is far lower now, due to decent housing and sanitation, improved perinatal care, the discovery of antibiotics and other medical advances. Life expectation is the biblical three score years and ten, plus a bit more besides. Fewer deaths take place in the home nowadays, less than one in three. Consequently, it is quite possible to go through life without ever seeing a dead person or giving the subject of death any serious thought. The obsession of the film and television industry with violent death furthers this avoidance, portraying death as something so glamorous and horrific that viewers are prevented from perceiving it as a reality at all. It is easy to understand, when one adds to the present degree of unfamiliarity with death the amount of fear which any mention of the subject can arouse, how the death taboo came into being.

When a fatal illness is diagnosed, or a chronic illness reaches its terminal phase, many doctors recoil from the prospect of involvement in the patient's future care. Their training has often prepared them for a curative role only, and an imminent death may feel like an assault on their self-image. The feelings of failure, fear and impotence frequently prevent them from filling the vital and demanding role which is left open to them. Nursing staff are often equally ill-prepared for the task of caring for a dying patient. Although their sense of failure may not be so acute, their inability to avoid close contact with the patient when providing basic physical care can lead to intense emotional discomfort.

The extent of the taboo on death can rarely be seen more clearly than when someone dies in certain hospital wards. Although aware that a patient has only a few days or hours left to live, every effort is made to act as though this were not the case. Inappropriate treatments, such as intravenous feeding, and the recording of irrelevant observations, such as the blood pressure or urine output, are continued to the very end. Fellow patients showing concern about the obvious deterioration in the dying person's condition are frequently rebuffed. They may receive loud and clear messages that it is none of their concern, or their intelligence may be insulted by the pretence that everything is going to be fine. Even when a death has occurred, it is not customary to inform other patients. Evasion and even deception are common. The awareness of a death by fellow patients only becomes apparent at visiting times, when it is possible to hear whispered information being passed on to relatives and friends.

Often it is felt more appropriate to nurse a dying patient in a single room. There are all manner of justifications for this: less noise, less bustle, more privacy and so forth. However, it can also be a very satisfactory means of reducing to a minimum everyone's discomfort concerning the dying patient.

After death, the body is removed from sight as quickly as possible. Once the plugging, packaging and labelling are completed, it is whisked away to the mortuary in a box specially designed to look like an ordinary hospital trolley, whilst the nursing staff go to extraordinary ends to ensure that no one sees it. Unfortunately, the sound of the mortuary trolley seems to arouse even more fear when all sight of it is obscured. The dead person's belongings and any evidence that he was once in the ward are removed behind closed curtains, with all possible speed. Within minutes, a freshly made up bed replaces that of the deceased, great sighs of relief, and hey presto, everyone is buzzing around again as though nothing had happened.

So, not only may thought about death be avoided, and those who are dying be kept at the furthest distance possible, but also their death may be virtually ignored. In addition, there has been a decline in the rituals which have traditionally encouraged the mourning process, whereas most of those which have been retained guarantee a further period of protection from reality. It is no longer customary to allow the dead body to lie at home, for this practice would force the family into an acknowledgement of the reality of the death. Instead, it is taken to an undertaker's, where it may later be viewed in the chapel of rest. In North America, where death denial is carried to its furthest extreme, funeral parlours are a lucrative concern. The body is embalmed and dressed in a favourite outfit, and great cosmetic and hairdressing skills are employed to make the corpse look as life-like as possible. A piece of chiffon-type material is usually placed over the face to further protect the viewer from any slight remaining semblance of death. Visiting and viewing the body are conducted in an impersonal and institutionalised way. All instinct to touch and embrace the body and to weep over it at length whilst saying goodbye is inhibited.

The funeral service will often say nothing personal about the one who has died. This may even be a conscious decision to avoid evoking any unnecessary distress. The Jewish and Roman Catholic faiths forbid the coffin to be left open during the service and it is certainly not encouraged by many Protestant denominations.

Once death is over, the newly bereaved and those who had nursed the dead person are left to continue the game of pretence; pretence that nothing of any great significance has occurred.

Chapter 2

The Hospice Movement

The care of the dying has been undertaken by religious orders for several hundred years. A hospice was originally the name given to a place of rest for pilgrims, and it seems fitting that this name is being used for the centres which are springing up all over the world to provide a resting place for those in need of peace and care in the last stage of their journey through life.

Until the opening of St Christopher's Hospice in London in 1967, deaths took place in general hospital wards, at home, in private nursing homes or in one of the few convent hospices, such as St Joseph's Hospice in Hackney, run by nursing nuns. With the notable exception of the convents, the care given in these various places was usually the best that could be provided in the circumstances, amidst the demands of busy wards and with the limited knowledge of symptom control that was available. Even when the patient was nursed in his own home it was frequently far from satisfactory. Here, the family doctors and community nurses were often unable to relieve the patient's suffering. Some would experience feelings of guilt and inadequacy, but others failed to recognise their deficiency or did not think it important. The advances in medical technology seemed to do nothing to improve the care of the dying and, in fact, sometimes made hospitals even more unsuitable places in which to be cared for.

Dr Cicely Saunders, who was first a nurse and then an almoner before qualifying as a doctor, was more aware than most of the inadequate care provided for the dying. After seven years spent working with the nuns at St Joseph's, she gathered together a group of people to help raise the money to build another hospice. Her aim was to create an environment in which patients and their families would be able to adjust emotionally and spiritually to approaching death, much as she had seen at St Joseph's. At the same time, she aimed to develop ways of relieving the pain and other distressing symptoms experienced by the terminally ill in a more scientific manner. The result of this was the opening of St

Christopher's Hospice; because of the pioneering work done there, a network of hospices now exists throughout the world. (For details of hospices in the UK, see 'Hospice Information', page 202.)

In 1974, the first British unit providing hospice-type care within the National Health Service was opened at Christchurch, near Bournemouth, in the grounds of a general hospital. Eighteen months later, similar units were opened in Oxford and Southampton and, since then many more have been opened within the National Health Service. The capital cost of these buildings has been met by the community in which they are situated, as the result of appeals launched locally by the National Society for Cancer Relief. On completion, they have been handed over to the district health authority, which has then provided the revenue costs.

There are many other independent hospices like St Christopher's: these include St Luke's Nursing Home in Sheffield, several Marie Curie Memorial Foundation Homes and a few Sue Ryder Homes. Although not under the auspices of the National Health Service, between fifty and seventy-five per cent of their running costs usually comes from the health authority concerned in the form of contractual beds. Even though this arrangement can be very satisfactory, providing both the majority of the finance as well as a degree of freedom, those units on general hospital sites also have many advantages. Hospice values and standards of care are seen to be essential and integral components of the health service, rather than optional extras. The easy access to radiotherapy treatment, X-rays, the surgical treatment of fractures, pharmacies and central sterile supplies are but a few of the many practical advantages. The staff have the advantage of working in a less isolated atmosphere, with a constant exchange of information with staff from other departments.

WHO BECOME HOSPICE PATIENTS?

The great majority of hospice patients, approximately eighty per cent, are suffering from some form of malignant disease, even though these are only responsible for one fifth of all deaths in the Western world. In most other cases death is either very sudden, or else curative treatment is continued right up until the moment of death. In malignant disease, however, there is usually a very definite and often lengthy period at the end of the illness when active treatment aimed at cure has been discontinued. Even palliative treatment aimed at controlling the disease or holding it in its current state of advancement may have to be abandoned, since the time will frequently come when the side-effects of the drugs or radiotherapy will be as dangerous to life as the disease itself. For these reasons, a large number of patients who are classified as 'terminally ill' and are, therefore, eligible for admission to a hospice, will be suffering from some form of malignancy.

Other patients who are sometimes cared for in hospices are those in the terminal stage of degenerative neurological diseases, such as multiple sclerosis and motor neurone disease. There is no reason why any dying patient should not be cared for in a hospice, but those who have been patients of a particular hospital department for many years, suffering from chronic obstructive airways disease or renal failure, for example, may prefer to be cared for by familiar staff in familiar surroundings. Nevertheless, it is important that hospice care is always regarded as an option, and one that will provide the best care for some patients.

Since hospice beds are scarce, selection of those patients in greatest need must sometimes be very stringent. Priority is usually given to younger patients in whom both mental and physical suffering is often more severe and whose social needs, particularly when young children are involved, can be immense. Priority is also given to those with intractable pain or other unrelieved symptoms, and those who have no one to care for them at home. Short-term admissions are often arranged for symptom control or to give relatives a break.

HOME VERSUS HOSPITAL

Everyone involved in hospice work is agreed that home is the right place to die, if this is the patient's choice and circumstances make it possible. The surroundings are safe and familiar, and the family, if there is one, can rally together to provide the very best care. Relatives, friends and neighbours can visit more easily and remain closely involved, whilst the fear and loneliness of hospital are avoided.

In hospital, many people experience feelings of anonymity. The sense of belonging, of having a role to play in which one feels useful and valued, and the sense of personal identity are far easier to maintain at home than in an institution, however enlightened it may be. When death is approaching, one of the strongest feelings is often that of loss of control, but so long as it is possible to remain in one's own home, some semblance of control can be maintained.

However, home care may not always be possible for many reasons. These include social isolation, exhausted relatives, intractable pain, the need for frequent dressings or other nursing procedures, the inadequacy of domiciliary services (such as home helps, night nurses or laundry service), or inadequate housing. With sufficient motivation and knowledge some of these difficulties can be overcome, but so much will depend on the key relative or friend. Some will be physically frail and therefore unable to cope, whilst others will be so distressed by incontinence or a colostomy, for example, that they are emotionally incapable. Where a relationship has been unhappy for a long time, home care may be undesirable to both patient and carer.

Sadly, most families have become so adjusted to the institutionalisation of death, that one is often working against their wishes when encouraging home care. Many patients request hospital admission, either because they want the security of medically qualified staff around them, or because they do not wish to be a burden on their friends and relatives. When confronted with families who are terrified of the death occurring at home, and a patient who is asking to be cared for in hospital, it may well be too late to attempt to change attitudes and there is no alternative but to respect their wishes.

HOSPICE VERSUS HOSPITAL

The advantages of hospice-type care, when compared with the care which can be given in a general hospital ward, are many. The staff have chosen to care specifically for dying patients, and their motivation will therefore be far stronger than in those for whom this is a necessary, though not particularly desirable, part of their work. The concentration on terminal care leads to a far greater expertise, particularly in areas of emotional support and symptom control. The conflict between the needs of the acutely ill and the terminally ill patient does not arise. There are no pre-meds to give, drips to watch, or, with rare exceptions, patients to be prepared for the operating theatre, and there is certainly not the same speedy turnover of patients found on a general ward. Although the nurse-to-patient ratio is usually the same, the basic nursing care can always take priority and it can be done at the patient's own pace. The staff are a stable team, usually containing a large element of older nursing auxiliaries who seem ideally suited to this type of work. The fact that the majority of the staff are not in training and are, therefore, not moving from ward to ward, creates an increased sense of security and continuity for the patients. The homeliness of the environment, the air of peace, and the involvement and care of relatives are all possible to some degree on a general ward, but they are certainly much easier to achieve in a specialist unit.

However, hospices or terminal care units also have some disadvantages. Even with small bays containing two to six beds, some of the slightly longer-stay patients are likely to experience anything up to ten deaths during the length of their admission. In this age of unfamiliarity with death, there is no doubt that witnessing a peaceful death can be of great comfort to many people, but to spend the last weeks of one's life continually developing relationships with other patients, then watching them die, one after the other, can be a most distressing experience. Most people would prefer to see life and living around them at this time, not perpetual death and mourning. Some patients on general wards are distressed by the fact that everyone else is recovering and going home, whilst they alone are getting weaker, but even this may be preferable to witnessing so much death. Some staff working in this field have a tendency to be blinkered by their idealism. So great is their concentration on caring for the patients that distress caused by the environment often goes unrecognised. They forget how different it feels, wandering in and out of a room containing patients near to death when one is ambulant, involved in providing practical care and going off duty at the end of an eight hour shift, compared with the feelings of those who are bed-bound amidst dying people for twenty-four hours a day. To those unfamiliar with illness and death, the stertorous, irregular respirations of a dying patient can seem quite terrifying in the dark of the night, and not all deaths appear peaceful and dignified to the onlooker, even when the dying person himself is not suffering. Since most patients will be aware of the imminence of their own death, every unpleasant symptom observed in fellow patients who are dying is likely to be interpreted as a possible future threat to the onlooker.

Another disadvantage of the specialist unit is the fear and anxiety aroused in patients when told that they are to be sent to one. In many cases, no one has previously had the courage to discuss the patient's prognosis with him. Imagine his feelings then, when told he is to go to the hospice, well-known in the area as 'the death house' or 'the place you never come out of alive'. However, even these criticisms cannot negate the tremendous contribution of hospice work. One has only to see the effect which this type of care can have on both the patients and their families, and hear what they have to say about it, to be convinced of its value.

THE FUTURE OF THE HOSPICE MOVEMENT

The aims for future development appear to point in three directions.

HOSPICES

The first is the provision of a small, hospice-type unit in each major town and city. Such a unit would not attempt to mastermind the management of all dying patients, but rather serve as a pool of expertise for community and hospital staff to draw from, as well as filling a teaching role, particularly in the training of doctors, nurses, social workers and ministers of religion. In-patient care would only be provided in cases of extreme need, where the expertise of specialists was really necessary. Ideally, a patient would be admitted to a self-contained flatlet which would also accommodate his immediate family. This would enable family life to continue, allow the relatives to continue to provide much of the care, and avoid exposure to constant deaths.

HOME CARE TEAMS

The second aim would be the development of domiciliary services to advise and support the community staff, as well as providing an extra tier of care for the patients and their families where this is needed. Many home care teams are already functioning, but this is an area where further expansion would be of the greatest value.

Where a domiciliary team is available, not only is the quality of care improved, but some patients who would otherwise have been admitted to hospital are able to die at home. The team usually includes several nurses with a health visiting or district nursing background as well as experience in hospice work. Other staff involved are generally doctors, social workers, occupational therapists and chaplains, who are also working within a hospice. Most domiciliary teams work from a hospice base. Although a few have been established independently, usually within a community nursing division, and have provided a valuable service, most have felt the need to have some hospice beds available as a safety net.

The domiciliary nurse is not normally involved in the physical aspects of nursing care. Because the nature and size of her caseload is so different from that of the district nurse, her visits can be longer and a greater depth of involvement is often possible. She reviews all symptoms and the adequacy of medication frequently, informing the general practitioner of any change. She also reviews the nursing needs and, where appropriate, offers advice to the district nurses or enlists the help of other agencies. But perhaps her most important role is the provision of emotional support for both patient and carers. She has the willingness, the ability and the time to listen. Occasionally, she is called upon to advise or explain, but by far the greatest part of her time is spent listening. Little may be achieved if district nurses see this work as a threat to their own role and relationship with the patient. But if the domiciliary nurse is sensitive to the feelings of the district nurse, and if both value the contribution of the other, their combined efforts can result in a very high standard of care.

Where a home care team is based in a hospice, there are three other ways in which their support can be developed. The first is the establishment of a 'sitting service'. This consists of a pool of trained nurses, as well as other unqualified but suitable people, who can be called upon to sit with patients in their own homes, particularly at night, in order to give relatives a rest. The second is the provision of a day hospital (see page 11), and the third is a 'medical loan service', to ensure that any item of equipment needed by a patient at home can be supplied immediately.

The final role of the home care team is the support of the bereaved. This usually takes the form of home visiting, but may also include group meetings, when members of the home care team invite several bereaved relatives to attend a social gathering. Great support can be gained by sharing experiences with others in a similar position, and valuable friendships are sometimes established. Where a suitably qualified social worker or psychiatrist is available, more formal group therapy may be provided. Some relatives would find none of these forms of help desirable or appropriate, and few would be helped by all three. It is, therefore, apparent that they should be offered with great sensitivity.

HOSPITAL SUPPORT TEAMS

The third and final aim would be the formation of hospital-based support teams. These would be multi-disciplinary groups, taking the expertise of specialist units onto the general wards; advising and supporting staff when they have dying patients in their care, and again, providing an extra tier of care for patients and their families. Since far more patients die in hospital than either in hospices or at home, it seems essential that any expertise in this field is channelled into the general wards as soon as possible.

A few such groups are already in existence, some of which call themselves 'symptom control teams'. This title is more acceptable to many nurses and doctors, since it conforms with their view of medicine as being concerned, primarily, with physical problems. Although the members of these teams do not see their role in any way limited to controlling symptoms, they are prepared to live with this title, since their consequent acceptability increases patient referrals.

The main function of some of the earlier hospices was to admit dying patients in order to care for them during the final phase of their illness. In many units this work has evolved, developing in the three areas just described, and some new units which are opening have these aims in mind from the outset. However, there are still some hospices, both old and new, which limit their work to in-patient care during the final stage of the illness.

CONTINUING CARE UNITS

Some of the newer hospices call themselves 'continuing care' units. This is not necessarily a euphemism, although it is a term which most patients and their families find more acceptable than 'hospice' or 'terminal care home'. Patients are referred to these continuing care units as soon as curative treatment has been discontinued, sometimes sooner. They may require an initial admission for assessment, symptom control and emotional support. Alternatively, this may be provided in their own home by the domiciliary staff, or on a general ward by the unit's support team. Intermittent admissions, possibly one week in four, or even three days a week, may be necessary to reassess symptoms and adjust medication, or just to keep the patient's morale intact. The intermittent admission may also be essential for the sake of the relative who is providing the care at home. Without this help, they may eventually collapse from exhaustion, thus necessitating permanent admission for the patient.

Many continuing care units provide the facilities of a day centre for patients being cared for at home. The average attendance varies from once to three times a week. In this way an opportunity can be provided for socialising, for physical nursing care such as baths or dressings, for physiotherapy and occupational therapy, for entertainment, for hairdressing, and for medical examination with an assessment of symptom control. Meanwhile, the relative has the benefit of a few hours 'off duty'.

Patients who are able to remain at home throughout their terminal illness and who do not attend the day centre will see the hospice doctor as an out-patient. With this degree of support, many patients are able to spend the majority of time in their own home during their final weeks of life. Most are able to die at home, if they wish to do so. Admissions very close to the time of death are actively discouraged. The arrival of moribund patients can be very distressing to those who then have to nurse them, and death occurring within a few hours of admission can leave relatives with a great deal of guilt. But both of these disadvantages pale into insignificance when compared with the lack of humanity that a last-minute admission expresses towards the patient.

After the patient has died, the unit's home care team will continue to support the family through their bereavement, often for as long as two years after the death.

The use of the term 'continuing care' does seem to be justifiable, although it sometimes leads to confusion with units providing rehabilitation or care for the chronic sick.

A large number of deaths, particularly amongst those occurring in the elderly, are quiet, peaceful affairs, often taking place at home with minimal preceding illness. But, unfortunately, this is not always the case. Many of the dying require a great deal of help. To keep a dying person mobile and mentally alert, whilst controlling his sometimes vast array of symptoms, demands a lot of time, commitment and expert knowledge. To provide the emotional support needed by such a patient and his family makes further and no less taxing demands. But the time, commitment and expert help are not available in many wards and general practices.

Even now, only about one person in a hundred dying in Britain has the support of a hospice, a home care team or a hospital support team. It is essential that the expertise of these specialist groups should not be so narrowly restricted, and that it should become available to all those working with dying patients in general nursing and medicine.

Chapter 3

The General Philosophy of Caring for the Dying

The underlying aim of terminal care is to help people to die well, in comfort and with dignity. This can only be achieved if the needs of the body, mind and soul are met in unison. It is essential to create an atmosphere in which adjustment to forthcoming death can be encouraged and helped, but this will be of little value if severe physical pain is meanwhile left untreated. Similarly, pain-relieving drugs will be less effective, however skilfully used, if they are prescribed in a cold and indifferent manner; hence the need to treat the whole patient. But even this is not enough. The very highest standards of care may be achieved in vain, unless every aspect is tailored to the needs of the individual patient and family.

THE VALUE OF INDIVIDUALITY

Every patient encountered has a unique personality, social background and experience of life. Time and effort spent getting to know the whole person and developing a relationship with him is always well spent. Not only does caring for the patient become infinitely more satisfying, but also very much more effective. This may sound too elementary to be worth mentioning, but the infrequency with which it is implemented warrants its reiteration. It is the recognition of this individuality which is the corner-stone of good terminal care. Physical symptoms must be treated with such skill that the patient is kept comfortable, whilst remaining mentally as lucid as possible. Only in this way will he be able to retain his individuality, to stay 'in charge', and to live what time remains to him in his own way.

In hospital, as in any other institution, there is a great temptation to treat people in a uniform manner within the framework of a highly organised routine. This may make for the most smooth-running and tidiest of wards, but it does not in any way value or respect the individuality of the patient, without whom there would be no ward or nursing staff. It may seem extremely inconvenient to have to help someone with a bath at nine o'clock in the evening when all baths are usually taken in the morning; it may seem an absolute nonsense making a separate pot of tea for someone who likes their own fancy China variety; it may seem like the last straw getting someone to bed at midnight when their friends have just brought them back from an evening out, but this is the price of individualised care.

Our sense of our own individuality is greatly enhanced by our possessions and our clothes. Patients in hospital can gain great comfort from surrounding themselves with those items which hold particular significance or value, such as pictures, books, photographs or a work-basket. Because this is not traditionally acceptable, permission and encouragement to do so will be necessary. Pyjamas or nightdresses and dressing gowns worn during the daytime do little for the patient's morale. Permission and encouragement will again be needed to wear ordinary day clothes. Many patients find this more normal mode of dress very reassuring. The use of hospital clothing is best avoided whenever possible, even if this means washing the patient's own clothes for them. Few things increase the feeling of anonymity more than wearing someone else's clothes.

Those who have undertaken a hospital training, in which some degree of regimentation was necessarily the norm, will have to get over a huge psychological hurdle in order to see this whole matter in perspective. Patient-centred care comes as second nature to many nursing auxiliaries, who have not been moulded by a hospital training, and it is a return to this more instinctive manner of caring that must be achieved. All manner of objections will immediately spring to mind whenever patient-centred care is contemplated, the most common being the shortage of time. When people are dying, the very least we can give them is a little extra of our time, though this may not even be necessary once we have cut out the unnecessary recording of routine observations such as the temperature, pulse and respirations, the blood pressure or fluid balance, and have accepted the help of willing relatives.

When meeting a terminally ill patient for the first time, the nurse should take a biography rather than a medical history. As much as possible should be learnt about the patient's past, about his work, his interests and his family. Few people will reject this attempt to get to know them and most will be delighted and grateful. A full hour will usually be about the right amount of time for the first interview, although it will vary widely. A shy, apprehensive patient may become very anxious about such a lengthy interview, whilst the more garrulous may chatter away for an hour before getting anywhere near to discussing the matters of real concern. Physical examination to assess the condition of pressure areas, the skin, the mouth or any dressed lesions, for example, and the recording of relevant medical history and current medical details are, of course, essential. But if they can be prevented from dominating the proceedings, the patient is far more likely to feel respected and cared for and less like the 'malignant melanoma in bed number 12'. This whole approach is becoming far more widespread with the arrival of the 'nursing process', since the latter advocates a similarly individualised style.

Hospitals must of course be as cost-effective as possible, and this is partly achieved by a high level of bed occupancy. Nevertheless, it is not reasonable to sacrifice quality of care for quantity. Whilst it would be perfectly acceptable to reallocate the bed of someone who was admitted for the extraction of wisdom teeth within minutes of discharge, it would not be acceptable after a patient had just died. What would neighbouring patients assume about the staff's attitude towards the deceased, if this were the case? And more importantly, how valued would they feel themselves, since they would be likely to identify strongly with the patient who died? Surely the price of a bed left empty for twenty-four hours is not too costly a means of showing respect for the dead? An occasional emergency admission, when no other bed is available, may be unavoidable, but this could be the exception rather than the rule.

Many of these suggestions for more individualised care sound like those things which are only possible in a private nursing home, not on a busy National Health Service ward. However, when caring for terminally ill patients, it is essential that nursing priorities are reorganised. Since many of the aspects of care vital for acutely ill patients become superfluous, time can be reallocated more appropriately.

RECOGNITION OF FAMILY AND FRIENDS AS KEY MEMBERS OF THE CARING TEAM

In caring for the whole patient, one is also caring for those people closely involved with him. Seeing that a companion or spouse is receiving the care and practical support that they require will do as much for the patient's peace of mind as any care directed at him personally. Unless relatives are enabled to maintain their involvement as key members of the caring team, the quality of patient care will be greatly depleted. When a patient is being looked after at home, the key role played by the family or friends with whom he lives is self-evident. This role tends to blur into the background in hospital, unless the staff take positive action to prevent it from happening.

The relationships which develop between dying patients and members of the health care team can be deep and valuable, but, in the great majority of cases, these play a subsidiary role to the relationships with family and friends. In the small hours of the night, when so many fears come out of hiding, it is the familiar presence of a trusted friend or relative that affords the greatest comfort and reassurance.

When a patient is admitted to hospital, if the next-of-kin has accompanied them, they too will need to be 'admitted' in the sense of an admission interview. While the doctor or nurse is taking a biography from the patient, another member of staff can take the next-of-kin into a private room and spend some time getting to know him.

It is very useful to hear an account of the patient's illness from the relative at this point. Such a sharing will not only be of practical value to the nurse, but will also be therapeutic for the relative. They will very often choose to reveal information about financial or relationship problems within the family, which may have great significance for the future care of the patient. Their knowledge of the patient's likes and dislikes, dietary habits or special ways of relieving pain should be recorded in a notebook. This will reassure the relative that his information is not only valued and respected, but that it is also going to be implemented.

The relative will no doubt be feeling extremely 'emotional' during this interview. It is not suprising that, when the attention previously focussed on the patient is redirected onto the relative himself, simply by enquiring after his well-being, the result frequently resembles the opening of a floodgate. With encouragement and support, the tears may flow for five or ten minutes.

Hospital admissions are almost invariably surrounded by guilt on the part of relatives, who feel that they have failed their loved ones. They may also feel guilty about the relief they are experiencing, and these feelings will often be heightened by the exhaustion of weeks without adequate sleep. They will need to share these feelings both in words and in tears, and they will need to be validated repeatedly for the tremendous job that they have done in nursing their relative for so long at home. Remarks about how well cared for the patient looks will mean a great deal to them, as will reassurance about the inevitability of the admission to hospital.

During a prolonged illness, some of the grieving which usually occurs during bereavement takes place whilst the patient is still alive. Apart from grief at the anticipated loss, there will be a great deal of anxiety about the future. How will she manage financially? How is he going to cope with two young children as well as his job? Not every close relationship is a good and loving one, and when there has been much bitterness and pain, the combination of grief at the imminent death, and guilt about the sense of relief it brings, can be a terrible burden for anyone to carry alone.

It is important to bear in mind that the relative's feelings about his own mortality and death will have been aroused by the patient, and help may be needed for him to be able to acknowledge and express these. Simple questions, such as 'Have you ever been close to someone dying before?', or 'What were you most afraid of when you were caring for your sister at home?', will often be all that is needed to initiate such a sharing.

It is apparent from this small selection of emotions, all of which are commonly experienced by relatives at such a time, that the potential for skilled counselling during the 'admission' interview is enormous. (See page 56 for a description of counselling.) The trust that is established at this first meeting is crucial, since it is likely to flavour all future relationships between the relative and members of the staff.

In addition to meeting the relative's own need for comfort and support, it is at this early stage that he should become aware that he is still recognised as the key member of the caring team, thus maintaining his close involvement and consequent feeling of value. This can be done by involvement in making decisions on nursing and medical management, by a constant sharing of information about the patient's condition, and by telling him how good his support has been and how greatly the patient values him and needs his support to continue. Passing on complimentary and loving remarks that patients have made to members of staff about their relatives is very important, especially if they are the kind of people who would never pay each other compliments first hand. Care must be taken, however, never to breach confidentiality.

One other useful way of maintaining the relative's role in hospital is by encouragement to participate in the care of the patient. Involving relatives in the physical aspects of nursing care is not always a labour-saving or a time-saving activity. In fact, the initial task of teaching the relative how to perform the care, and the support needed to develop their confidence in the early days, may make additional rather than diminished demands on the staff. It is helpful to accept this from the outset, and to acknowledge that the value to both relative and patient is the prime motivation. Nevertheless, some relatives, after an initial break to recuperate when the patient first comes into hospital, will once again take on all the basic nursing care required during the daytime, lightening the nurse's work-load considerably. A good night's sleep each night, plus the support of the staff, may enable them to continue to be the main agent of care, and this will be the best care possible for the patient. It may also help to prevent feelings of worthlessness and uselessness from occurring in the relative and the possibility of self-recrimination during bereavement. Less confident relatives may not want to be involved in the same way, but they can be encouraged to refill the water jug, plump up the pillows, or to assist in the serving of meals and drinks. Their presence should be welcomed when the patient is, for example, being bathed, dressed or helped into bed. In this way, they can often be made to feel that they are being useful. The somewhat prudish practice of asking a husband or wife to leave the bedside at such times can be extremely hurtful.

Because nurses are always in a care-giving role, while patients and their relatives are on the receiving end, it is very easy for the former to assume, quite unintentionally, an attitude of authority. In their misguided attempts to support and protect those for whom they are caring, they frequently take over responsibilities and decision-making in a quite unacceptable manner. The nurse's role is to support the relative, so that they are better able to cope with their own responsibilities, but not to take them over.

QUALITY OF LIFE, NOT QUANTITY

Too often, those close to death are kept alive or are resuscitated without any consideration for their wishes or for the quality of life which remains. This applies equally to younger patients suffering from a fatal disease as it does to elderly, debilitated patients who develop a potentially fatal illness. The most extreme, but not particularly unusual, example of the latter is the severely demented patient in his eighties or nineties who is no longer able to communicate, lies permanently curled up in a foetal position with his eyes closed, who is doubly incontinent, has bed sores and severe contractures which are almost certainly painful. On developing a chest infection, instead of allowing nature to take its course, parenteral antibiotics are administered.

Many more people are living into old age nowadays than ever before, and it is becoming increasingly difficult to find the resources, financial and human, to provide adequate care for them. Since this problem is certain to continue growing, it seems even more important that those who no longer find their quality of life acceptable should be allowed to die naturally. Death must be seen as an acceptable part of life, not as a medical failure. Much of the attention at present focussed on saving life at all cost would be more appropriately channelled into the provision of better care for the dying, thus improving the quality of the life that remains.

Those who know that their life is limited by a fatal illness, and are unfamiliar with the course it is likely to take, will frequently seek advice from their doctor, health visitor or community nurse about how much they can do, and whether or not some things are dangerous. It is essential that these professionals should enlist the help of family and friends in encouraging the patient to live whatever life is left to the fullest possible extent. Anxious and protective relatives must be discouraged from pampering and smothering the patient. They must be gently helped to understand that such behaviour will merely succeed in reinforcing the patient's view of himself as an invalid and a burden. They will need to have accepted the inevitability of the death before they are able to stand by whilst the patient takes risks.

Risks are part of the very essence of life for the terminally ill. If they were to avoid all actions which might precipitate a worsening of their condition, the quality of the life that remained could be so poor that a slight increase in quantity would be irrelevant. It is essential, however, that both the patient and those close to him are prepared for any likely crises. They need to know what actions may precipitate an untoward happening, and precisely what to do if it should occur. To impart this information clearly, but in such a way that anxiety and unduly protective behaviour are decreased, rather than aroused, demands a great deal of the nurse or doctor concerned. It is only possible when the patient is treated with the respect of an equal, when his right to receive such information, and his right to decide how to use it, are recognised.

Many patients with malignant disease have metastatic deposits in their bones. When these are painless, walking should be encouraged, although if they are sited in the hips or legs, this may well mean risking a pathological fracture. Should this occur, pinning the fracture, analgesics and bed rest will almost certainly relieve any pain which is caused. Even then, little is lost, but several months more of freedom to walk about independently is the likely bonus.

Those with relatives on the other side of the globe may have a great desire to visit them for the last time. Concern about possible haemorrhages, fits or sudden demise should be discounted. Never mind if the climate is damp and cold. How much better to die of pneumonia five thousand miles from home, with the joy of having seen a much loved son, of having held an only grandchild for the first time, or having visited a long unseen and much-yearned-for friend, than to live a month longer, sad and lonely. Trips to the theatre, country walks, picnics, parties or a drink at the local may well leave the patient exhausted. He may even have to stay in bed for the whole of the following day to recuperate. This is no problem at all as long as he recovers in time for the next evening's activities.

Nothing whatsoever will be gained by restricting a dying person's food, alcohol or tobacco consumption. So many patients with lung cancer spend their last weeks gasping for a cigarette, which they feel too ashamed or nervous to smoke. Those whose disease has been treated with steroids are especially likely to have problems with obesity due to a ferocious appetite. What can be gained by putting them through the trauma of a reducing diet, and who has the right to put a heavy drinker through the distressing symptoms of alcohol withdrawal? Any hint of disapproval of these so-called vices from nursing or medical staff can cause tremendous unhappiness, whilst a glimmer of acceptance can alleviate much of the shame and guilt. This seems a very small indulgence to ask of even the most ardent teetotaller or anti-smoker.

Very few people enjoy being treated and regarded as invalids, especially when their days are numbered. To obtain the maximum quality of life, rehabilitation should be the aim of treatment right until the very last lap of the disease. The housewife who is able to maintain her role by planning the meals, writing out shopping lists, organising a family rota for cleaning, washing and ironing, even if she is not able to do any physical work herself, will feel a far greater sense of usefulness and belonging than if her role were taken away from her completely. Many household tasks, such as preparing vegetables, paying bills or polishing the silver, can be done from an armchair or even sitting up in bed.

During the last days of life, many patients feel that all they have left to offer their families is their love and their thinking. So often, in an attempt to care for the patient, relatives overprotect them to the extent that they feel unable to give even these. Patients invariably sense when some cause for anxiety in the family is being kept from them, and they feel hurt and resentful at being excluded and prevented from contributing their support and concern. Moving the patient's bed into the living room can often help to avoid this feeling of exclusion. Although welcomed by the patient, this may be discouraged by the family, however, since the containment of the patient in an upstairs bedroom is often part of the relatives' mechanism for coping. Whilst the patient is out of sight, it is possible to deny the reality of their dying and continue living normally. But if their bed is moved downstairs, the relative is constantly confronted by the pain of reality. The district nurse is often the best person to help relatives to understand how lonely and isolated the patient is feeling, to support them in looking at and dealing with their need for denial, and to help them in their adjustment if the decision to move the patient is made. In the days when many houses had servants, and direct contact between patient and relative did not necessarily occur, it was not uncommon for relatives to avoid seeing the dying person at all during the last weeks or months of their life.

With adequate analgesia, some severely ill patients are able to continue in their normal job of work until a few days before their death. There may be an element of denial in this determination to carry on working as normal, but better a bit of denial than the feeling of worthlessness experienced by so many overprotected and pampered patients.

It is important not to forget the small minority of patients who simply love being helpless, having everything done for them and who totally abdicate all their responsibilities. It is often very difficult in hospital to give these patients the pampering and care that they demand. This is partly because of the pressure of work and partly because the staff will understandably resent these demands when far weaker patients are struggling to maintain their independence. Friction will invariably occur. Patients who fall into this group are often very unhappy people, desperate to be loved and cared for, because they have suffered from a lack of affection during their lifetime. They are one category of potential 'unpopular patients' and, as such, are considered more fully later in this chapter.

ADAPTING THE HOSPITAL ENVIRONMENT
PEACE AND QUIET
A relaxed atmosphere is essential for the peace of mind of a terminally ill patient. Unnecessary noise and bustle should be avoided at all costs. On

a busy general surgical or radiotherapy ward, this may be quite impossible to achieve. However, with thought and care, noise and bustle can almost always be reduced significantly, particularly at night, though it does take considerably longer to perform a task quietly. The introduction of admission wards is a great boon here. Many dying patients are able to detach themselves from, or even sometimes enjoy the activity going on around them, but they are greatly distressed if their own care is perfunctory and hurried. Because they are so weak they are also very slow, and any attempt to make them do things more quickly will leave them feeling flustered and out of control. On a general ward, it is often far better to delay the patient's blanket bath and dressing until the least pressurised time of day, when it can be done in a more leisurely manner.

The nurse who appears calm and relaxed inspires trust and confidence. One of the great arts of nursing is the ability to work quickly and thoroughly, whilst appearing to have all the time in the world.

DOMESTICITY

Many patients are unnerved by the clinical unfamiliarity of a hospital ward. Anything which makes for a more domestic atmosphere will be of value in helping them to feel more at ease. Open visiting will ensure that a few friends and relatives are about almost all of the time, which not only makes the ward feel more homely, but the tension and noise caused by set visiting hours are avoided. However, for the patient's sake, it may be valuable to introduce an afternoon rest period, and staff will need to be especially observant to ensure that those patients receiving large numbers of visitors do not get unduly fatigued. A quiet word in the ear of a close relative may be necessary if this does happen, since patients themselves should not have to cope with the difficult task of turning visitors away, or asking for visits to be kept brief. Needless to say, it is the patient's feelings on this matter which should dictate such action, rather than the nurse's judgement. It may be necessary to teach some relatives how to use their visiting time. So often they feel obliged to engage the patient in continuous conversation, which is quite alien to their normal pattern of relating. This can be harrowing for the patient and can cause a great deal of tension in the visitor. They should be encouraged to behave as they would at home, sitting quietly knitting, reading the paper, or watching television together.

Nothing does more to make the hospital feel a relaxed and homely place to be than the freedom for children of all ages to visit. They have remarkably little fear of very ill patients, often being quite oblivious of their jaundiced or emaciated appearance. The sight of a toddler clambering over his grandfather's bed will bring delight to most patients. It is often the visit of young children, who talk so uninhibitedly to all the patients around, which breaks down the barriers of reserve between patients. Few children are rowdy enough to cause irritation to anyone in this situation.

It is easy to underestimate the importance of pets in many people's lives. It may sound unhygienic and eccentric to suggest that pets be allowed to visit, but it can transform a hospital admission for many patients, especially those who have lived alone, to have their life's companion brought in to see them. A well-trained dog will often lie quietly for an hour on his master's bed, causing no trouble to anyone. Obviously there is a need for great discretion, but the possibility should not be overlooked.

For the patient who is still ambulant, freedom to make himself a pot of tea or a piece of toast, as and when he feels like it, will help him to retain some semblance of the autonomy he would have in his own home. The value of this feeling far outweighs the possible danger of scalds or burns, the reason so often given for disallowing such fundamental activities.

BEAUTY

People vary widely in the way they respond to their visual surroundings. Some appear to be almost oblivious, whilst those with an artistic nature can be affected profoundly. When dying patients are bed-bound, it is particularly important for nursing staff to be sensitive to their aesthetic needs. Tape recorders, radios and talking books can all be used with earphones, making literature and music of all kinds easily accessible. The responsibility for visual beauty in hospital will, however, fall largely on the nursing team.

The decor is very important. Garish colour schemes should be avoided in favour of warm and gentle shades. The clinical appearance of stark, white hospital bedspreads can be overcome by individual bed-squares, crocheted by patients, relatives or local women's groups. If this is done, it may be a good idea to suggest a colour scheme to prevent too gaudy a collection. Carpeted floors not only look nicer than the traditional shiny surface, but are warmer, quieter underfoot and feel more homely. Many patients will welcome an invitation to have one of their favourite pictures brought in and hung where they can see it.

It is a good idea for all nurses to take the opportunity of lying on an empty hospital bed and sitting in a bedside chair occasionally, to remind themselves of what patients can and cannot see. Flowers are so often placed where everyone but the patient himself can enjoy them. Plants and flowers can do so much to enhance the appearance of a hospital ward, but quite the opposite when they are neglected. This is an area where the help of patients, visitors or volunteers can be useful.

Bed-bound patients should always be given priority over those who are ambulant when allocating beds with a window view. No dying patient should be condemned to spend the last days of his life gazing at a blank wall. Trees, shrubs and bird tables can provide a feast for the eyes and souls of many patients.

Some 'hospital smells' are unavoidable, but it is worth remembering that it is these smells which evoke fear and repulsion in so many people. The unnecessary use of antiseptics should be avoided whenever soap and water would be as effective. Nurses have a tendency to try to drown unpleasant smells with more acceptable ones, but unfortunately the combination of the two is often worse than the original malodour. Fresh air is usually the best antidote if draughts can be avoided.

The sense of touch is sometimes a source of extreme pleasure to dying patients. A cushion covered with a cool satin material or a warm, soft velvet may bring great comfort. Although the exhaustion caused by most fatal illness seems to dull aesthetic sensitivity, in some cases the reverse occurs and there is a heightening of awareness and appreciation of beauty.

INFORMALITY

Informality is the final aim in creating the atmosphere most conducive to the patient's ease and sense of belonging. The value of informality is in the removal of barriers which arise between patients and those caring for them. It has often been claimed that any such loss of professional distancing would cause a concurrent decline in standards of care. However, it would seem far more likely that the depth and quality of the care would improve with the dropping of those barriers, and that the use of professional formality is a means of protection from any real involvement. There is no room for self-protection in caring for the dying. Patients need befriending above all else, and this means becoming closely involved, getting to care deeply for them, sharing the pain of their suffering and grieving at their death. There will be reciprocity in such a relationship. Patients will usually enjoy hearing about the families and social lives of members of staff, so long as this is kept in proportion to the amount of attention given to them and only divulged at the patient's request.

There seems little value in the use of hard and fast rules about the manner in which patients are addressed. Some, particularly those in the older age groups, would feel that they were being treated quite disrespectfully if anything other than their formal title were used, whereas most younger patients appear to feel far more comfortable when addressed by their first names. However, if the use of first names were the norm enforced upon the ward by the staff, few patients would risk future unpopularity by objecting. Great sensitivity is obviously required. Informality between members of staff is also an important factor in creating the general atmosphere. Their use of first names amongst themselves can be a very valuable leveller. Patients who pick this up and address the staff informally are obviously more at ease in doing so. The aim is to make it easy for patients to use whichever form comes most naturally, without pressure either way.

PROVISION OF EMOTIONAL SUPPORT

The pivot around which the whole philosophy of the care of the dying revolves is the acceptance of the whole person. There is no room for judgement, criticism or a desire to change or convert. All that is required is willingness to meet and accept the person in the condition that nature and nurture have rendered them. Every human relationship demands this same element of acceptance, but for those in the last stage of their lives it is especially important, for if it is withheld until the person is deemed worthy, it may be too late. Complete acceptance will embrace both tolerance and respect. Without these, a relationship of trust will not develop, and without trust, effective support is not possible.

During a terminal illness, patients and relatives are certain to be experiencing some of the most painful emotions. These commonly include fear, frustration, guilt, grief and anger. Suppression of emotions such as these will not make them disappear. Until they have been allowed to surface and to hurt, they will be lurking about in the subconscious, often causing both emotional disturbance and physical ailments. It is a great deal easier to focus on painful thoughts and experience the pain which they arouse, when someone else is there to share it and offer support. It is hard to stay close to someone who is expressing strong, negative emotions, but this is the nurse's most vital contribution. It will usually be most effective when a counselling model is used (see page 56).

Some patients and relatives are able to use their families and friends for this purpose, but many have no one with whom they feel sufficiently safe. Members of the caring team must, therefore, be ready and able to fill this role.

When painful thoughts are shared, strong emotion may be vented and this should be welcomed and encouraged. The patient or relative will need to be told continually how well they are doing and should experience no sense of rejection or withdrawal of affection. Dying patients should not be expected to remain in a permanent state of composure. The human body was created with its own inbuilt healing system for dealing with emotional distress, just as it has a physical healing system for dealing with injuries and infection. However, one of the peculiarities of our society is that, right from childhood, people are discouraged from using this healing system. A child who is releasing feelings of sadnes when a favourite toy is broken soon has his tears quelled by the soothing adult, hence his sadness is suppressed. Little boys, in particular, are encouraged to cultivate a 'stiff upper lip' from a very early age. Similar means are employed when anger is expressed in a raging temper tantrum, fear by trembling, or embarrassment in giggling. By the time we reach adulthood, the ability to use these natural methods of emotional release has usually been well and truly eroded by the belief that it is undesirable. Only within a relationship of mutual acceptance, openness and trust will it feel safe enough to rediscover and utilise this system of healing.

In order to meet the patient's emotional needs, in addition to developing a relationship of trust and a willingness to stay close, there must also be an understanding by the carer of the psychological stages which people experience in approaching death (see Chapter 4).

It is impossible to provide emotional support for the dying unless one is strongly motivated. Many doctors and nurses find it a particularly unwelcome part of their workload, which they carry out with distaste and a lack of enthusiasm. An enormous personal commitment is essential. The trust in the relationship is a two-way phenomenon, for in order to give of herself to the extent that is needed, the person in the caring role will become exposed and vulnerable. Patient and carer will enhance each other's humanness in this state of mutual trust and openness, and grow together.

There are many practical ways in which nurses can provide emotional support. The patient who requires hospital admission will need reassurance that his arrival was expected, that the staff know something of his condition, and that he is welcome. A guided tour of the ward, with particular emphasis on lavatories, the patient-call system, quiet rooms, public telephones and the areas where smoking is permitted, can help to reduce anxiety. Introductions to fellow patients and a few members of staff are also important. It is particularly helpful if the care of a newly admitted patient can be allocated, for the first few days, to the nurse who conducted the admission interview. Some patients will need to be told that the welcome will remain even if they do not show signs of recovering. They may need reassuring that discharge home will not be considered unless they make considerable progress, or they may need a guarantee that discharge will be organised just as soon as their symptoms are controlled.

Within the unfamiliarity of a hospital environment, the importance of recognising the patient's need for his 'own space' is vital. The position of his bed should not be changed unless absolutely essential, and only then with the patient's consent. Respect for his need for privacy is another major concern in an open ward. The use of curtains around the bed should be offered and encouraged – many patients are reluctant to use them unprompted for fear of offending their neighbours.

The patient being cared for at home may need reassurance about the availability of a hospital bed if the situation at home breaks down, and a guarantee that his pain will be controlled adequately wherever he is cared for.

Patients with foul-smelling and disfiguring tumours need extra special reassurance of their total acceptance. Physical contact is particularly valuable in conveying this message. This can take the form of a handshake on first meeting; as the relationship deepens it may be the offer of an arm when walking to the bathroom, an arm around the shoulder if the patient is distressed, or sitting quietly at the bedside of someone very weak, holding their hand. The manner in which nursing treatments are performed can also relate messages of acceptance or rejection (see page 176).

Although the sexual drive of a very ill patient will almost always be greatly reduced, their need for physical contact and the comfort derived from it may well be greater than usual. It can provide closeness, prevent avoidance and relieve both guilt and jealousy. A sensitive nurse can help enormously in relieving the patient's embarrassment by offering the privacy of a single room, whenever possible, and ensuring that visits by partners are not disturbed unnecessarily. If the partner is staying in hospital with the patient, provision for them to sleep in the same room is essential, however cramped. Hopefully, the day will come when hospital side-wards are equipped with double beds. A great deal of misery is frequently caused by abstinence from sexual closeness. This is often a result of the relative's fear of harming the patient, the patient's fear of causing repulsion by their diseased body, and both their feelings that sexual desire is inappropriate when someone is terminally ill. When nurses are willing, and sufficiently confident to encourage the sharing of such anxieties, a great deal of misunderstanding is sometimes unravelled and feelings of isolation avoided.

The relatives of a patient who is brain-damaged and who has become sexually uninhibited will need tremendous compassion, understanding and commonsense advice to cope with his behaviour. Such a patient may expose himself or masturbate in an open ward, causing great embarrassment to other patients and their relatives, as well as those visiting the patient himself. Although the use of a single room is obviously one solution, the nursing staff must take care not to reject and neglect such a patient, and visitors should not be left unsupported with him for long periods. Everyone on the ward will need help to understand that this behaviour is out of the patient's control, and nursing staff will need to exhibit great care and watchfulness to protect his dignity.

Physical pain cannot always be totally relieved, but the patient who feels accepted and cared for and has confidence in those looking after him is usually well able to cope with any residual discomfort. Likewise, the patient who lacks this confidence and feeling of care and acceptance may interpret every symptom as a threat to his survival and will often magnify them out of all recognition.

POPULARISING THE UNPOPULAR PATIENT

WHO ARE THE UNPOPULAR PATIENTS?

Wherever ill people are being cared for, whether in institutions or in their own homes, there will be a certain number in their midst who get labelled as difficult or unpopular. They may be considered as such for one or more of the following reasons.

The first group of unpopular patients consists of those who have some major social difference from those who are looking after them, though their behaviour is, in fact, quite normal within their own society. This will include people of a different colour, race, faith or class. It is a sad fact that the unfamiliar and apparently strange habits of those from a different culture will frequently evoke hostility. This may be partly due to insecurity caused by unfamiliarity, particularly when there is a language barrier, but it may equally be due to in-built prejudices. The heavy drinking, infested tramp is just as likely to arouse this prejudice as a wealthy sheik or a punk rocker.

Middle-class patients, who appear to be demanding the standards and trappings of private care in a National Health Service setting, will rapidly gain the disapproval of many a working-class nurse. Their accent alone may be sufficient to evoke hostility. Demands for a single room often grate, especially when these are used to continue running a business, to obtain privacy for entertaining, or to hold a complete library so that work on a thesis can continue. This prejudice may be heightened by the increased friendliness and extra attention of the middle-class doctor towards these particular patients and the contrast of the very low demands of the working-class patients. Similarly, staff may well feel threatened by the more intelligent patient, who demands detailed information about his treatment. This is especially likely to provoke ill-feeling if the member of staff is inadequately informed and the patient clearly knows more about his own case than they do.

The fact that almost all forms of prejudice are understandable does not mean that they are excusable. Those who nurse dying patients have a special responsibility to be aware of their own prejudices and to overcome them, or at least to try not to act on them. If this is not achieved it will be impossible to meet the dying person's emotional needs.

The second group of unpopular patients contains those whose behaviour makes them difficult to like. It could be that they seem totally unaware of the plight and needs of the other patients in the ward, thinking only of themselves and demanding immediate gratification of their every whim. Attention may be demanded in quantities far exceeding the average, often at the expense of other patients. Alternatively, they may be uncooperative, refusing treatment which is offered for their own comfort and well-being. Others will gain unpopularity because their symptoms do not respond to any of the treatments which have been carefully thought out and conscientiously applied.

Everyone in a caring role, however well motivated they may be, needs some recognition of their individuality by those for whom they are caring. This need not involve the sharing of detailed accounts of their personal lives but does, at least, need to constitute an awareness of their individual existence. Being addressed by one's own name, e.g. Sister Green or Dr Tyler, is so much more endearing than 'nurse' or 'doctor'. Patients to whom one nurse is just the same as the next are very difficult to care for, since the provision of care is dependent on the formation of a one-to-one relationship.

Those who are unappreciative, unhappy or unattractive are also amongst those likely to be labelled as difficult patients. It is easy to see why staff frequently avoid patients displaying difficult behaviour, preferring to spend their time with the quiet, grateful, cooperative and cheerful patient who shows thoughtfulness about the staff and the other patients. However, it is the difficult patient who really needs the time. A difficult patient is one whose needs have not been met. In caring for the dying, many staff find themselves able to exempt even the most infuriating patients from judgement. Instead, they provide all the extra attention and tolerance which the patients demand. The change which this uncritical care can bring about is sometimes quite dramatic. Those who seemed so egotistical and who demanded constant attention may, after several weeks of receiving the kind of care that they need, make minimal demands on the staff, spending much of their time attending to the needs of other patients.

WHY ARE SOME PATIENTS DIFFICULT AND HOW CAN THEY BE HELPED?

In order to facilitate the provision of such care, it is useful to understand why some patients behave in a difficult way. The majority of emotional development takes place during early childhood, and the most important ingredient at that time is the feeling of being loved and wanted by those around. A child who is rejected by his mother or mother-substitute may well grow up emotionally stunted in his capacity to respond to, and accept, affection from other people. Children who are overprotected may remain permanently emotionally immature. They often become shy, withdrawn adults who retain a high level of dependency. A combination of rejection and overprotection may lead to a lack of self-confidence and an inability to trust other people. Although personality development starts with the genetic inheritance of characteristics, maturation may never occur without the right emotional environment to nurture its growth. The contribution of other influences and experiences towards development will be minimal. It is rather like an oak tree growing in a plant pot; however much fertiliser and nutrition is provided, the growth remains stunted.

With independence and health, much of the damage caused by early emotional deprivation can be superficially camouflaged. However, with the fear, anxiety and insecurity aroused by a fatal illness, it is not surprising that the effects of this damage become apparent. It is rarely appropriate at this stage to launch into full-scale psychoanalysis or psychotherapy. This would aim at unravelling the early causes of the damage and working on the feelings which have long since been repressed. It is a lengthy procedure which often makes the patient feel a great deal worse before he starts to feel better. The time factor rarely makes this feasible in terminal care. Instead, psychiatric expertise may be enlisted to help in a patching-up procedure. More often, a high degree of acceptance, tolerance and respect from the whole caring team will be the best treatment possible.

There is always a temptation to withdraw from relationships which prove unrewarding, but by avoiding difficult patients their behaviour is likely to be made even more difficult. It may take an enormous effort to keep relating to and sticking close to an unpopular patient, but if he is to be helped at all, this will be essential.

RECOGNITION OF SPIRITUAL NEEDS

Simply coping with the day-to-day physical and emotional demands of a terminal illness seems to sap every drop of energy from many dying patients, leaving little attention for higher thoughts. Those for whom religion played no significant role during their lifetime rarely experience an upsurge of religious thought and interest when dying. Similarly, concern with philosophical questions and the existence of an afterlife is uncommon in those with no previous tendency to explore these areas.

And yet, surely everyone has spiritual needs of some kind, particularly those who are approaching death, whether or not they aspire to a specific faith and whether or not their needs are expressed in religious terms. Death raises some of the deepest questions about the meaning of life and about man's relationship with himself, with others, and with the universe.

Those involved in the care of the dying need to recognise that living in a pluralistic society, they are likely to come into contact with a wide variety of faiths and beliefs. Barriers of prejudice are likely to arise as a result of ignorance about, and unfamiliarity with, many of these faiths and their associated customs. To overcome them, it is helpful to familiarise oneself with the basic concepts of the more common belief systems. But it is far more useful to find out from the patient himself exactly what his beliefs are, because the beliefs of the individual may differ widely from those generally accepted within his particular faith. In a sharing of thoughts such as this, the real spiritual needs are most likely to emerge.

Christianity, being the predominant religion in the West, is likely to colour the perception of spiritual needs and the way in which it is thought that they should be met. Because of the subservience of the laity in most Christian denominations, the majority of spiritual needs are passed over to the priest or chaplain, particularly where the priest is believed to have an exclusive, God-given role as mediator. This seems both sad and unnecessary. Whatever the religion or belief, there can only be one truth, for believers and non-believers alike. If this is the case, everyone should take confidence in their own ability to give and to gain spiritual support in any situation. This in no way denies the role of the ministers of religion, but ensures that others are able to make their contribution. In addition, the needs of the patient can be met at the time they are voiced by the person to whom they are addressed. A pastoral counselling session on the following day may be of little value.

No audience is more captive and more vulnerable than terminally ill patients occupying hospital beds. For this reason, members of staff have a vital responsibility to respect and protect them, taking great care never to abuse their position by imposing their own beliefs upon patients uninvited, however fervently evangelistic their own faith may be. Too often, patients will accept this as the price they have to pay for the care they are receiving.

The nursing staff should also be aware of evangelising doctors, clergymen and fellow-patients, being quick to notice when anyone is feeling uncomfortable or lacks the confidence necessary to handle a situation. When this happens, if the patient so wishes, nurses may be called upon to intervene. Although demonstrating sensitivity and respect for the motives and beliefs of the evangelist, the patient's interests must be her prime concern. The nurse may also find herself supporting colleagues who are feeling guilt about their failure to convert someone before they died. This can be a dangerous attitude in anyone working exclusively with those who are terminally ill, dangerous both to themselves and to the patients for whom they care.

It is often the task of the nurse to inform the appropriate minister of religion when someone is seriously ill and to enlist his help in supporting the patient and those close to them. Timidity in this area is frequently shown when help is needed for a Jewish, Hindu, Buddhist or Muslim patient, largely because of unfamiliarity with both the faith and with the members of the community concerned. A non-believer may even feel reluctant to approach the Christian ministers of religion for the same reason. The sooner that relationships are established with these people, and an interest and concern shown about their particular faith, the sooner will they feel able to share their knowledge and skills with the nursing staff. The hospital chaplain will usually know the whereabouts of all local religious communities and will be able to provide details for contacting their ministers or leaders.

It can be disastrous to ask a minister of religion for help just when a patient is dying. The appearance of an unfamiliar person, who has quite obviously been summoned because death is imminent, will not surprisingly seem sinister and frightening to many patients, especially if they are at all confused or if they had never practised the faith to which they were nominally ascribed. Involvement at the earliest possible stage is the obvious answer, not least because the patient is then able to decide for himself whether or not this is desirable.

The patient who has had minimal previous contact with his religious minister may feel ill at ease and unsure of how to relate to him when receiving a visit in hospital. If nursing and medical staff are seen to be relating to him in a relaxed and welcoming manner, the patient will feel more able to do likewise. If staff seem unfriendly or indifferent, however, the patient's embarrassment may be heightened. Ministers of religion and representatives of religious communities have an invaluable role to play in the care of dying patients, but they can only fulfil this role if they are included in the caring team. It is vital that everyone involved in the care works in a united way. Professional jealousy or prejudice bar open communication. Information should be shared freely and support extended to every member of the team. This includes, of course, the ministers of religion, who otherwise can easily become isolated.

PASTORAL COUNSELLING

The main function of the pastoral counsellor, whether he is the rabbi, the doctor, the next-door neighbour or the nurse, is the development of a relationship with the patient which enables the sharing of thoughts and feelings, and offers help in dealing with them. All manner of spiritual concerns may need exploring together; issues commonly raised at this time are thoughts about life after death, euthanasia, the relationship between sin and suffering, man's purpose in life, and how to tell children about death. The best advice for a nurse in this situation is not to try to provide the answers. There probably are none, but even if there are, the only relevant ones are those that the patient works out for himself.

The anger which may be felt at the imminent loss of one's own life is difficult to express without a target. If someone believes in God, this clearly is where the anger is likely to be directed, but many people are afraid to admit to feelings of anger with God and need a great deal of support to do so. The counsellor must find a means of demonstrating that the release of anger is acceptable to God, and that there need be no fear of retribution. The Christian may gain comfort from being reminded of the cry attributed to Jesus when he was dying on the cross, 'My God, my God, why hast thou forsaken me?'. The release of such anger may prevent it from being turned inwards and causing a self-destructive depression. (See also pages 68–70).

Many patients looking back over their lives are only able to focus on their times of weakness or apparent failure. Such memories can make the approaching death more painful to contemplate. The pastoral counsellor will enable the dying patient to review his life in a more positive way. Explanations for failures will be found, and attention will be focussed on the times of happiness, growth and fulfilment. With this more rounded summing up of his life, the patient may approach death at greater peace with himself.

RELIGIOUS PRACTICES

It would be unforgivable if religious doctrines appertaining to either a dying or dead person were not adhered to at all times. These vary widely from one faith to another.

For the dying patient who is a Christian, there are many forms of worship which can be made available. These include the sacraments, in particular confession and absolution, Holy Communion and the annointing of the sick. Some patients in hospital will wish to participate in communal worship, but others will prefer to hear Bible readings or prayers said at their bedside. These are unfamiliar to many people, however, and need offering sensitively after a relationship has been established with the priest concerned. (There are some exceptions to this norm. Many Roman Catholics will greatly appreciate sacraments given by a most unpopular or previously unknown priest, due to their perception of his role.) Even in the fulfilment of these more specific services, the presence of the priest is not always essential, unless the sacraments are being administered. Lay parishioners who are particular friends of the dying person should feel able to say prayers at a patient's bedside, and most nurses, Christian or agnostic, would feel happy to read a patient's favourite passage or psalm from the Bible to him when he was too weak to read for himself. When Holy Communion is being administered or prayers are being said, it is important that curtains are pulled around the bed to provide privacy and to protect other patients from any embarrassment this might cause.

Patients in hospital may find silent meditation very difficult in an open ward. A hospital chapel is almost always available, and even those patients not strong enough to walk can be taken in a wheelchair or on their bed. It is important that no one is deprived of this type of prayer when they are dying. For the Christian, it may be the time when they are most receptive and open to God's love. Great strength and comfort may be lost if silent meditation is not possible. A rapidly increasing number of non-Christians are now practising various forms of meditation and they too will have the same need for peace and quiet. The knowledge that a busy nurse is standing by, waiting for the meditation to end so that she can whisk the patient back to the ward and so resume her work, is guaranteed to inhibit the meditator. Nurses should be prepared to allow patients an agreed amount of time without surveillance, however ill they are, if this is their wish.

Ward prayers said in the morning or evening can give great comfort to many patients. Those who are non-believers, or who are of a different faith, are rarely offended or distressed by this; in fact they, too, may gain comfort from the few moments of contemplation. Nevertheless, every patient should be consulted and given the choice to opt out if they wish to. The readings and prayers used need not always be specifically Christian. When someone known to be a Christian has just died, there is certainly a place for the use of commendatory prayers said kneeling at the bedside, joining hands with both the deceased and their loved ones. This act will help enormously in expressing a recognition of the profundity of what has occurred.

The anointing of the sick is available to Christians of several denominations, but it is particularly important to Roman Catholics when they are dying. This sacrament can be administered several times during a terminal illness. It may lead into confession and absolution, followed by a celebration of Holy Communion.

It is not mandatory for a priest to be present with a Catholic when he dies, though both the patient and his family will gain great comfort in most cases if this is possible. Roman Catholics are now at liberty to choose to be cremated.

Orthodox Jewish practice requires that every Jew is accompanied during his last hours of life, preferably by a rabbi, but otherwise by members of his own family, who will read a confessional service to him. There is a common Jewish custom of opening the windows immediately after a death has occured, to allow the spirit to escape. In hospital, the body may be taken to the mortuary, but cleansing will be carried out by members of a special Jewish burial society. Gentiles should not handle the body. During the time between death and burial, the body is often attended and read to from the Book of Psalms. Burial is mandatory and is always performed as soon as possible.

The last words that a Moslem should hear before he dies are the Islamic articles of faith in Allah. These are usually whispered quietly into his ear by family members. Moslems have very strict doctrines following death. The body is faced towards Mecca (i.e. in Britain towards the south east) with the head raised. Washing the body is very ritualised, certain parts being cleansed first and water splashed over it several times afterwards. A male may be washed only by another male Moslem or by a woman whom he could not have married, such as his mother or daughter. A female may only be washed by another female. Non-Moslems are forbidden to touch the body. Burial is compulsory, but no coffin is used.

A Buddhist is usually supported spiritually by a monk or priest when he is dying, preferably from the same school of Buddhism as himself. During the final hours he will recite the Sutra, bless the patient and ask him to recall his good deeds. Buddhists are encouraged to meditate for as long as they are able, resisting unconsciousness and remaining in a state of transcendency until the moment of death. The patient may also be shown a picture of the Buddha at this time. Because of the importance placed upon wakefulness, the taking of drugs which depress the central nervous system is discouraged. Afterwards, any funeral rites are considered to be grief therapy for the relatives.

Hindus are usually blessed by a priest when dying, and this may be symbolised by a thread tied around the neck or wrist. The priest pours water into the mouth of the corpse after death and the family then wash the body. Again, many Hindus prefer their deceased not to be touched by non-Hindus. Cremation is always performed as soon as possible.

Post-mortems are unacceptable to most Jews, Moslems and Hindus. If they are legally unavoidable, the relatives will be anxious that the organs are returned to the body before burial or cremation.

Priests, monks or nuns who belong to religious orders of any faith or denomination are usually attended by their fellow members, and are dressed in the vestments of the order once the last offices have been performed.

People of the same faith, but from different cultures and ethnic groups, will vary widely in their beliefs and rituals. Some will take a very liberal approach, adhering to few of their traditions, whilst others will wish to comply with every detail of their religious doctrine. It is important to obtain some understanding of a family's wishes well before the death occurs, whenever possible. If an interpreter is not readily available, the local council for community relations can usually help.

REFERENCE

Lamerton, R., *Religion and the Care of the Dying.* A Nursing Times Reprint. Macmillan Journals, 1973.

Chapter 4

Communication

The provision of care in any situation is dependent on effective communication. Communication is especially important when encountering or caring for someone who is dying, but it is also especially difficult. The fit person is frequently experiencing great emotional distress, feelings of pity, grief, revulsion and helplessness. The encounter will often be fraught with fear. The dying person is afraid of his disease and of the future. He may also be afraid of what he is going to hear and of the distress he sees his presence can arouse. He is afraid of being isolated and alienated. Deep-rooted fears of illness and dying may also surface in the fit person. It is not surprising, therefore, that communication with people who are dying is, in general, not very effective.

It is important to remember that dying patients are perfectly normal people who just happen to be dying sooner rather than later. The survival instinct will always encourage us to regard them as a breed apart, thus pushing away the reminder of our own mortality. This feeling of difference or separation can form a barrier to communication.

THE NURSE'S ROLE

Worries about saying the 'wrong thing' are often prevalent in those caring for the terminally ill, not least amongst nurses. The dying person seems so vulnerable, and anyone who feels at all clumsy or inadequate in their relationship skills may be so afraid of hurting or upsetting them, that they shy away. The fear is often quite unfounded, but it is probably responsible for a great deal of distancing and scant communication. If there is sufficient trust and safety amongst the nursing team, role-play can be a useful tool for increasing both competence and confidence. Each nurse can benefit, not only from constructive criticism of her own performance, but also from observing the strengths and weaknesses of her colleagues' efforts. Debriefing after a role-play is very important. This is when the participants share the feelings they experienced when playing their role and switch back into being themselves again. If there is a medical social worker involved, she will often make the ideal leader for such an activity, since her training and expertise in communication is usually considerable.

The nurse's confidence in her ability to communicate well, and her ability to instil confidence, will be greatly influenced by the possession of certain information. She will need to be fully briefed about the patient's condition, medical and social, and about his present insight into his situation. She will also need to know the policy of the ward or unit about revealing diagnostic or prognostic information. This can vary widely. Some doctors feel that no one, including themselves, should discuss these topics openly with the patient. Some will insist on being the only one to discuss the matter. Others will insist on being the first to broach the subject but, thereafter, permit the social worker and nurses to play their part. Others again will permit only certain nurses, usually the ward or community sister, to discuss these matters. Fortunately, many doctors, including those involved in hospice work, believe in a more liberal, team approach. They discuss every case openly with the nursing staff so that no inaccurate or presumptive information may be passed on. It is then left to the patient to select the member of staff he wishes to talk to about his situation. After an interaction in which the patient reveals progress or change in his awareness of his situation, his permission is usually sought to feed this back to the team. Some units use a special 'insight' page for recording this information in the medical notes.

It should be mentioned that doctors are not alone in preserving the less liberal approaches to this type of communication. Many nurses are unwilling to participate, fearing the extra responsibility and depth of involvement. It is also fair to say that most patients expect their doctors to be the ones who give them information about the severity of their disease, while expecting the nursing staff to add clarification and to help them to work out the implications. Nevertheless, some patients, particularly the less articulate and those overwhelmed by fear, may never have the courage to ask their doctor for information, but may well ask the district nurse, in the privacy of their own home, or the student nurse, during the intimacy of a blanket bath. If the freedom to talk openly in these situations is prohibited, those patients in greatest need of emotional support may be denied it.

When nursing a dying patient for the first time, anxiety and a feeling of inadequacy are almost inevitable. With experience, these feelings usually lessen and the confidence to communicate openly and spontaneously increases. The inexperienced may gain skill and confidence from being 'a fly on the wall' when more experienced colleagues are talking with patients or their relatives. Although unlikely to learn a great deal from the content of the interaction, observing the manner in which it is conducted can be valuable. What is said by the carer is of minimal importance. What really matters is the feeling behind it, which the patient will sense, and the ability to listen. Listening to patients or relatives should never be seen as a passive activity. The quality of listening which is needed demands every last drop of attention and empathy.

Nevertheless, it is as well to remember that however vital good communication with members of the caring team may be, it is the communication between patients and their families and friends which really matters. Any help given to facilitate the latter is the most valuable contribution any member of the team can make.

TIME AND PRIVACY

Most members of the caring professions, particularly nurses and doctors, find it all too easy to hide behind the cloak of busyness. Good communication does take a great deal of time, but how many of the tasks that we fit into our working day are really much less important? Both patients and relatives need to know that we are prepared to give them the time that they need. This is communicated instantly by our manner.

The district nurse who bustles in, rushes through a blanket bath and dressing at a rate of knots, chattering cheerily away throughout, is saying quite clearly that she has no time to listen. The family doctor who never visits his terminally ill patients unless specially requested to do so, and when he does, keeps his coat on, rarely lifts his eyes from his prescription pad and leaves the house in five minutes flat, is giving the same message.

It happens with even greater frequency in hospital, when the consultant, complete with his entourage of students, housemen and registrars performs his ward round. Animated discussions take place around each bedside. Admittedly, the patient often feels his own presence to be somewhat superfluous amidst the exchange of incomprehensible medical details but, nevertheless, he senses their commitment to his case. However, when the ward round reaches the dying patient, many consultants will merely acknowledge his presence by a courtesy greeting as they pass the foot of the bed. The rest of the team, following his lead, will either talk amongst themselves as they walk by, or else throw the patient an embarrassed, apologetic smile.

Nurses working in hospital cannot escape this criticism either. How high on their list of priorities do we find listening to patients? Even when the essential tasks of the day are completed, spare moments are so often devoted to reading up the notes, teaching sessions and ward cleaning. Of course these are all necessary, but so is listening. Ideally, certain periods of time should be allocated specifically for this purpose, so that the many nurses who still feel guilty unless 'doing something' are reassured that listening is an honourable pastime. There are still nurses in positions of authority who disagree with this view and never allow their juniors to sit down at a patient's bedside. Such detrimental values must be challenged, albeit courteously, and where no moderation can be achieved, taken to a higher level of nursing management. Occasionally, the restrictive practice of the 'dragon sister' proves to be non-existent. It is merely a projection of the nurse's reluctance to get too close to the patients.

One only has to sit down in an unhurried manner at a patient's bedside, or in an office or sitting room with a relative, allow eye-to-eye contact to occur and the message is given; you are prepared to give some time.

Privacy is equally important; few people will risk talking about things as intimate and potentially distressing as fears about their illness and dying in the middle of a busy out-patient clinic or ward. The use of curtains around beds, or even wheeling a bed into the privacy of a side-room, may be necessary. Ambulant patients are rather easier to take into the privacy of an interview room or office. At home, it may be necessary to be quite devious or bold to remove relatives from the room, in order to allow the patient to communicate more freely in a one-to-one relationship with their doctor or the district nurse.

CONVEYING INFORMATION

When information of a medical nature is being imparted to patients or relatives, it is always possible to adjust the mode of explanation to their individual knowledge and ability to understand. If this is done successfully, no one is insulted and no one is left baffled. It is, however, far simpler to use medical jargon in such a way that no lay person could possibly understand. This is the way in which a number of doctors opt out of communicating with their more seriously ill patients, often quite unconsciously.

All manner of defence mechanisms will leap into action if the information carries the implication of a poor prognosis or other distressing news, and neither relative nor patient will be able to understand fully or retain many of the facts. Information must therefore be disclosed gradually, allowing them time to mull over, absorb and raise questions about one aspect, before moving on to the next. It may be necessary to reiterate information several times over a period of weeks. It is salutary to bear this in mind before condemning our colleagues when patients claim to have been given no information at all. Anatomical diagrams are often a great help in conveying explanations, and their tangibility seems to give great comfort. Similarly, instructions about treatments, or the meaning of certain medical words or terms, can seem far less frightening if written out on a piece of paper and given to the patient to keep. Much of this work will fall to the nurse, interpreting, clarifying and expanding on the facts given by the doctor. For this reason she must know precisely what the doctor has said. She must also be prepared to acknowledge the limitations of her own knowledge, never giving information about which she has any doubts.

The medical ethic concerning confidentiality demands that no one other than members of the health care team and the patient himself should be given information about his case. However, this is rarely observed once a fatal disease has been diagnosed. In fact, many doctors feel quite justified in divulging the full details of the diagnosis and prognosis to the relative, whilst giving the patient a falsely optimistic account, or blatant untruths, or sometimes no information at all. Any nurse who has earned the respect of her medical colleagues is in an excellent position to question and challenge this discrepancy.

It is clearly essential and proper that relatives are given information and are consulted on all matters of medical and nursing management, but this should be in addition to the patient receiving information, and not instead of it. Furthermore, relatives, like patients, should have the prognosis revealed to them in a sensitive, unhurried manner, since they too are likely to be devastated by its implications. So often, they have the full details thrust upon them at the time when the diagnosis is first made. It may come as a complete shock, in which case they will be far from ready to hear or cope with the full facts. At this time, relatives are frequently told either that they must or must not disclose this information to the patient, placing them under a tremendous and quite unjust strain. Conspiracies of silence which inhibit communication between so many terminally ill patients and their families can be initiated in this way.

The disclosure of information is not a 'one off' affair in the care of terminally ill patients. The channels of communication need to be kept open at all times so that frequent updating of information, reassurance and consultation are possible. It would be excellent if some of the impetus for this type of exchange could come from the medical and nursing staff. All too often it is the relative who requests to see someone who can give him the information he needs, and he frequently experiences great difficulty in obtaining it. Less articulate relatives who do not demand such an interview may receive no explanation of the case at all. Regular interviews with doctors, nurses and social workers should be the norm, and responsibility for arranging them should rest with these members of staff. Although not always feasible, it would protect many patients from deceit and many relatives from receiving information in a harsh, blunt manner if joint consultations were more common. In addition to these benefits, most patients and relatives would find it far easier to talk together after a joint interview than they would if they had both been seen separately.

Where several close friends or relatives are involved, it is sometimes difficult to decide to which person information about the patient should first be imparted, particularly when there is disharmony or competition between them. This happens most frequently when both a young spouse and the patient's parents are involved, or where a friend is closer to the patient than any of his relatives. Each case requires individual assessment, but whenever possible the family and close friends should be seen together. This will prevent the news from being relayed second-hand to anyone and may help to draw them closer together. The patient's permission should be obtained before divulging information to anyone and their wishes should be adhered to, even when the person they wish to be treated as such is not officially their next-of-kin. A great deal of tact and sensitivity will be needed, particularly in cases of marital separation and divorce.

The following piece of dialogue, and all the others included in this chapter, were scribbled down, as accurately as possible, immediately after each conversation had taken place. They are not intended as examples of 'how it should be done', since there is no right or wrong way, but simply as illustrations of the kind of communication which can occur between nurses and dying patients. Unfortunately, it is not possible to capture the atmosphere or feeling of a dialogue in a written account, and some of the words may seem rather cold and calculated, particularly without knowledge of the pre-existing relationships or evidence of the non-verbal component. It can only be hoped that they were experienced differently at the time, in the context of a caring relationship.

Hospitals are such familiar places to nurses that they can easily forget how frightening they seem to some patients and visitors. The following conversation confirms this point, demonstrating the patient's need to be kept constantly informed about what is happening around him. It also shows how, when given the necessary information, witnessing the death of a fellow patient can be a very positive experience.

Pulling up a chair and sitting down at Elsie's bedside

Sister: I just wanted to have a word with you about Miss C. (the patient in the bed opposite). I've noticed you watching her so anxiously and I know you had become such good friends.

Elsie: Oh, thank you, Sister, I've been so worried about her but I didn't like to ask how she was in case people thought I was being nosy. You know she hasn't woken up at all today and it's almost tea-time. She is going to wake up again, isn't she?

Sister: Well, it is possible that she may, but it's very unlikely, I'm afraid. She lost consciousness during the night, and the most likely thing to happen now is for her to stay like this for another day or two, until her heart and lungs fail and she dies.

Elsie: I thought as much. Do her family know?

Reached out for the Sister's hand

Sister: Yes, they do. In fact they have all known it was going to happen sooner or later for nearly three years.

Elsie: Did Miss C. know?

Sister: Yes, she knew too.

Elsie: Will she just stay peacefully asleep like she is now?

Sister: Almost certainly. She may get a bit restless, but I very much doubt it.

Elsie: When will you move her into another room?

Sister: We weren't planning to move her at all, but would you rather we did?

Elsie: What, not even when she dies?

Sister: Well, we certainly could do if you'd prefer it.

Elsie: I've never seen anyone die. What will happen exactly? She'll wake up then won't she?

Sister: No, she certainly won't wake up. You'll hardly notice she's died. Her breathing will get very irregular with long gaps between breaths. That sometimes goes on for twenty-four hours or more. Then, during the last few hours, the breathing gets very shallow until it just fades away. It's all very slow and gentle.

Elsie: Would someone sit with me when she's dying?

Sister: Yes, of course.

Elsie: In that case I think I'd rather you left her where she is. It seems awful to move her into a strange room. Besides I can keep an eye on her for you if she stays in here, and I can chat to her brother and sister-in-law. They have to visit separately because they've got kiddies at home, so they need a bit of company.

Pause

Do you mind if I ask something else which may sound nosy?

Sister: Please do.

Elsie: It's just that every couple of hours I see you or two other nurses pull the curtains around Miss C.'s bed for about ten minutes. Then I hear lots of movement and scuffling about. I just wondered what was happening.

Sister: Well, I'm not surprised you ask. It must seem very strange. In fact all we're doing is turning her over so that she doesn't get pressure sores. You notice next time. You'll see she's lying on a different side than she was before the curtains were drawn. We clean her mouth at the same time to keep it moist and comfortable, because she's no longer able to drink.

Elsie: Thank you so much for telling me all this. It really has put my mind at rest. I'd begun to wonder if anyone had even noticed. I feel so much better now. I know it's all under control.

Pause

If only I could go as peacefully as that. I know this wretched cancer's spread and I haven't got much longer, but my illness is quite different from hers, isn't it?

Sister: It is different, but there is absolutely no reason to suppose that when the time comes for you to die it won't be just as peaceful as Miss C.

Elsie: Do you mean that, honestly?

Sister: I do mean it, honestly.

USING THE TELEPHONE

It is customary for hospital telephone enquiries about patients to be answered in as brief and evasive a manner as possible. This seems unforgivable when skilled and caring telephone communication, particularly with the immediate family, can make such an enormous difference to their peace of mind. Rather than giving a pat answer about the patient's condition, how much better to find out who is telephoning. If you have met previously, tell them who is speaking and ask after their well-being; ask how they have slept and how their arthritis is today; ascertain when they last visited and give a detailed account of changes in the patient's condition since then; offer to pass on any messages to the patient and find out when they next plan to visit.

So often, a frail, elderly relative will have had to walk a considerable distance to the nearest public telephone. They may be desperately worried about their husband or wife, having previously been given inadequate information. They may be anxious about using the telephone if they are unfamiliar with it, their hearing may be poor and they may be distressed about being alone in their home. What consolation do they obtain from the usual curt reply, such as 'no change', 'quite satisfactory' or 'comfortable as can be expected'?

The following telephone conversation took place when an elderly wife telephoned to enquire about her husband, who had been admitted to hospital the previous day.

Sister: Norham Ward, can I help you?

Mrs K.: Can you tell me how Mr K. is this morning, please?

Sister: Yes, of course. Is that his wife speaking?

Mrs K.: Yes, I am Mrs K.

Sister: Oh, hello Mrs K. This is Sister speaking. Do you remember me? I am the one who took you up to the dining room when you brought your husband in to us yesterday.

Mrs K.: I know, I recognise your voice. You're the one with the dark blue uniform aren't you?

Sister: That's right. Well, your husband seems to have settled in very well. He slept right through the night and the pain in his leg is much easier this morning. We even persuaded him to eat some scrambled egg for his breakfast. I remembered you saying that he hadn't eaten a morsel of food for over a week, so I knew that you would be pleased about that.

Mrs K.: But he never eats breakfast, even when he is well.

Sister: Well, he must have built up quite an appetite by now. I expect it was the pain that was putting him off his food.

Mrs K.: Well, thank goodness he's eaten something. How long do you think he's going to be in hospital?

Sister: I can't really say yet, but if he stays as free of pain as he is now, I don't expect he will need to stay long at all.

Mrs K.: Well, I hope not. I shall be glad when he's home again.

Sister: Are you alone in the house?

Mrs K.: Yes, I am. I've never slept alone in a house in my life before. We've been married for fifty-six years and last night was the first night he's ever been away from me. I went into hospital when I had my gall bladder operation, mind you.

Sister: Are you a bit nervous in the house alone?

Mrs K.: I was last night. I kept hearing all sorts of noises. Nothing really, but I kept getting worried that there was someone in the house.

Sister: Did you manage to get any sleep at all?

Mrs K.: Oh yes. It was only during the evening that I got so silly. Doctor G. gave me some tablets last week because I had got so tired. I couldn't relax properly and go to sleep because I was worried that I wouldn't hear Bert if he called me. Anyway, they put me out like a light, so I slept like a log, even on my own last night. Is there anything my husband needs me to bring in for him?

Sister: Oh yes. He said he'd forgotten the tablets for soaking his false teeth in.

Mrs K.: Oh dear! I'll bring those in then and I'll bring him some fruit. Would he be allowed a Guinness if I brought him one in? He used to drink one every lunch-time.

Sister: That will be fine. It will do him good.

Mrs K.: How long do you think he's got, Sister?

Sister: I couldn't give you a definite time, Mrs K., because we really don't know how long it will be, but Doctor T. seemed to think it could be several months rather than just a few days, which I know was what you were prepared for.

Mrs K.: Really. Do you really think he might see another summer?

Sister: I think he may well do, but I should try to concentrate on enjoying the spring first.

Mrs K.: Oh Sister, thank you. If you could see how beautiful our garden is and how much work my Bert has put into it. you would understand why it is so important for him to enjoy another summer.

Sister: I heard him telling one of the nurses how to look after geraniums last evening, so I guessed he was a keen gardener.

Mrs K.: Well, I had better let you get on with your work.

Sister: That's all right. Can I give Mr K. any messages?

Mrs K.: Just give him my love and say I'll be in to see him tonight.

Sister: I'll do that. Have you got a lift?

Mrs K.: Yes, my son-in-law is bringing me in.

Sister: That's good. Well, I won't be here this evening, but if you want to know anything, do ask Staff Nurse Brown.

Mrs K.: Thank you very much. Goodbye Sister.

Sister: Goodbye Mrs K.

TO TELL, NOT TO TELL, OR WHAT TO TELL

The most controversial issue in any discussion regarding the care of the dying is the question of 'to tell or not to tell'. Of course, many deaths are sudden and unexpected, so it is only amongst those suffering from advanced chronic diseases, such as motor neurone disease, multiple sclerosis, renal failure or cor pulmonale, and those with advanced malignant disease, who are dying by inches, that the apparent imminence of death makes prognostic revelations a possibility.

But there can be no hard and fast rules in this matter; every patient and every family is unique and so must be the way in which they are given information about their diagnosis and prognosis. So many people are convinced that no one should ever be told the truth; and increasingly, too many people are becoming adamant that everyone should be told everything. It is unlikely that either end of this spectrum would often be appropriate.

Relatives often ask doctors and nurses not to reveal information to the patient, usually on the pretext that he would be unable to cope with it. This should not be regarded as binding, however, but rather as an indication that they too will need help to reach a position of mutually beneficial openness. Most relatives are sufficiently reassured if they are told that although the patient will not be lied to, he will not be confronted with any information he has not asked for.

Information should be given as and when the patient is ready to receive it, and he alone should dictate both the pace and the degree of openness. However, the majority of patients do appear to cope far better once they know the truth. Uncertainty can produce constant anxiety and inhibit psychological adjustment. Attempts to deceive are so often exposed at a later date and all confidence in the person concerned may be destroyed. In the majority of cases, the diagnosis will have been known to the patient since the very beginning of his illness. Even though it may not have been explicitly revealed to them, few patients fail to interpret lumps, weight loss, increasing weakness or radiotherapy, and even fewer will fail to pick up the non-verbal clues given by doctors, nurses and relatives. Anyone who imagines that it is possible to experience the symptoms and treatment of a terminal disease without any comprehension has either never been close to a dying person or else they are fooling themselves for their own comfort and protection.

Since it is so rare for patients to reach the terminal stage of their illness without a pretty sound idea of what is happening, it follows that few patients will need to ask 'What is wrong with me?', 'Is it cancer?', or 'Am I going to die?'. The real need is for high quality, caring attention, with plenty of time. Given these conditions, if a relationship of mutual trust and respect has been established, the patient will feel safe enough to share what he already knows, usually his diagnosis and the fact that he is going to die, but more importantly the painful feelings associated with this knowledge. This safety is not easily achieved, since some patients are overawed by doctors and nurses, and others will have been conditioned by earlier rebuffs never to raise these discomforting matters. In order to show that it is now permissible, but definitely not compulsory, open-ended questions can be asked. Examples are, 'You must be pretty worried about this illness of yours?', 'What have you been told about your illness?', or 'How are you feeling about things right now?'. These will encourage the patient who wishes to talk to do so, whilst enabling the patient who is not yet ready to talk, or who does not really feel safe with this particular nurse, to avoid doing so.

The questions that are most likely to be asked by patients are, 'How long have I got?', 'What should I expect in the weeks or days to come?', and 'What will it be like to die?'. Tremendous courage is required to ask these questions, but a great deal is also needed to answer them. It is essential to be sensitive to the feelings and expectations behind the questions. The patient asking 'How long?' may still be counting on another five years of life when, in fact, his prognosis is nearer five weeks; he may be thinking he is going to die any day when, in fact, it would be quite realistic to plan for another six months; he may be feeling desperate to know that there is an end in sight. A great many patients obtain enormous relief from being told that they will only have to put up with everything for a few weeks more. The only solution is that those in a position to reveal this type of information should know their patients well enough to be certain of their present understanding of the situation and their feelings about it.

Whatever the prognosis, it is never completely certain, and the patient's mental state can have an enormous effect in shortening or lengthening it. Patients should be given this information, and those who still have a will to live have a right to encouragement and support. They will need help to build themselves up physically with exercise and a nourishing diet as they exert all their strength in the fight for survival. The person who tries to encourage a dying patient to give in gracefully, when he is still full of fight, will meet with great enmity and resistance. This reinforces the necessity to treat each patient individually.

Some patients are desperate for an indication of the time factor. This may be for quite practical reasons connected with business affairs or finance. Even in these cases, the uncertainty should be emphasised and a wide margin of time suggested. The use of a phrase, such as 'months, rather than years' is far more acceptable than a rigid time limit such as 'two months'. Patients may appear to be demanding a hard and fast answer but, if this is given, all hope is destroyed and the patient is often overwhelmed by the knowledge.

Because many people reach middle age nowadays with no experience of death, a clear and truthful explanation of what to expect during the last days of their life is doubly important. Reassuring a patient that almost all of the pain he experiences will be relieved, that nothing will be done to prolong his dying, that he will almost certainly die in his sleep and that someone will be with him throughout, may do a great deal to alleviate his fears. But even reassurances such as these must be tailored to the individual. Some patients, after hearing that they will almost certainly die in their sleep, will be afraid of falling asleep again. In some instances, sharing what seems to be the most gruesome of information can be a comfort. A patient with faeculant vomiting and a grossly distended abdomen from small bowel obstruction may be much relieved by a careful explanation of the situation and how it will be managed. Nothing could be as horrific as he was imagining, 'that his belly would burst open' or 'that he would eventually vomit up his insides'. However, the same information which was such a comfort to one patient may terrify another.

Although it is probably clear by now that there can be no hard and fast rules about what to tell dying patients, there are three guiding principles which might be helpful. The first is to listen well. If we listen hard enough, the patient will tell us what he knows, what he wants to know and the pace at which he is able to work. The second is never to lie to patients. They have a right to the truth, whatever our assessment of their ability to cope. Although the pace at which the truth should be revealed will vary according to each patient's readiness to hear, there is never any place for dishonesty. The third is never to take away all possible hope. This again will be dictated by the patient. It may be hope for a miracle cure, hope for another remission, hope for a few weeks free of pain or hope for a life after death.

It should, perhaps, be mentioned here that dying patients and their families will not be needing to talk about dying all the time. Although the error is usually on the side of not allowing them to talk about it enough, the over-conscientious have, on occasions, been guilty of 'death and dying' their dying patients to death!

This next piece of dialogue began in a hospice day room, when a patient was being given his routine medication. He was dying from carcinoma of the bronchus and was admitted with severe pain from bony metastases. As far as his family, his general practitioner and his consultant oncologist knew, he had asked no questions whatsoever about his illness. It had proved extremely difficult to provide an adequate degree of pain control, but this was finally achieved by adding a potent anxiolytic drug to the existing regime of analgesics and steroids. This confirmed the view that anxiety was a major factor in exacerbating the pain.

Although the pain control was then good, the patient became extremely drowsy and unable to concentrate for more than a few minutes. It was generally felt by both medical and nursing staff that the pain was unlikely to diminish, allowing the drugs to be reduced, until he was able to find a way of expressing and sharing some of his feelings about his illness. Consequently, every possible opportunity to talk had been given, but every one had been rejected.

Sister: Your medicines, Arthur.

Arthur: Ugh, those again! What exactly are they?

Sister: Well, the white mixture is for the bony pain in your ribs and spine; the pink tablet is to reduce the inflammation in your lungs and make your breathing easier, and the clear one is a pain-killer for your chest pain, but it also stops you coughing as much.

Arthur: Mmm.

Sister: You don't sound very convinced. Aren't they helping?

Arthur: Yes, they help the pain a lot; in fact it goes completely some of the time, but I'm not taking any more of that 'jollop' I've decided.

Sister: Why's that, if they're really helping?

Arthur: 'Cos as long as I'm taking pain-killers, I don't know where I stand. Can you understand? I don't know if it's worse or better. Do you see what I'm getting at?

Sister: I think so. Do you mean that when you've got all your pain, even though it's so awful, at least you're in control? Whilst with the drugs masking your pain and also making you a bit woozy, you feel as though you're losing control.

Arthur: I suppose that's it. I'm not getting you into trouble with the doctors by not taking them, am I?

Sister: Of course not. I'd be in trouble if I were to force the medicine on you. But Arthur, knowing we can't get rid of the cause of your pain and knowing how bad it's been over the last few months, doesn't it seem best to lose a bit of control and lose the pain too?

Arthur: I don't know. To be honest, I'm bloody scared about not taking the drugs, 'cos I've forgotten how bad the pain was. I've been living on those pain-killers for over a month now. It's not only the pain though . . .

Long pause

Sister: What else scares you?

Arthur: Wondering what's really causing the pain, I suppose.

Sister: Have you ever felt like asking anyone about it?

Arthur: Well, I knew if I'd asked our family doctor he'd only fob me off with things he knew I wouldn't understand. I asked the wife though. I knew the Doctor would have told her if it was anything really serious.

Sister: What did she say?

Arthur: Just that I shouldn't worry so much, that I should be concentrating on getting myself fattened up and all that.

Sister: You believed her?

Arthur: I know when she's hedging; she never could keep a secret from me.

Sister: Did you press her?

Arthur: No. I knew she was only doing what she thought was for the best. You think you want to know the truth, but you don't really. Then worrying and worrying about it, lying in bed at night, that's the worst. Knowing the worst couldn't be as bad as that.

Sister: I'm sure that's right.

Arthur: Do you know what's really the matter with me, Sister?

Sister: Yes I do.

Arthur: Would you tell me straight?

Sister: Yes, I would, if I thought you really wanted to know.

Arthur: Well, I reckon it's about time.

Interruption caused by arrival of visitors

Sister: I tell you what. Grab hold of my arm and we'll walk back up to the bedrooms. If you're still sure you want to ask me when we get there, we'll go into the office where it's a bit more private.

Guided the Sister straight into the office and sat down

Arthur: It's lung cancer, isn't it?

Sister: How long have you known?

Arthur: Ever since I first went to the doctor, when my voice started getting husky and the coughing started. How long have I got Sister?

Sister: Thank goodness, that's one question no one can answer for you.

Arthur: Can't you give me any idea?

Sister: Well, I would say weeks, rather than days or years, but there's really no telling for sure.

Weeping now for the first time

Arthur: God, I'm scared. It's not dying that's so bad, but how it will happen. The pain's been so bad sometimes that I've longed to be dead time and time again over the last twelve months.

Sister: Arthur, I've never lied to you before and I'm not lying now. I promise that when the time comes it won't be nearly as bad as you're imagining. You'll just get very weak and gradually sleepy, not suddenly, but over a few days. The pain will almost certainly get less severe, it nearly always does, but if you have any pain, we can give you drugs to stop it. I promise that you won't die in pain and I promise that someone will be with you all the time.

Wept for five or ten minutes letting the Sister comfort him

Arthur: I shall have to tell my wife what you've told me, that it's cancer and everything.

Sister: As I think you'd guessed, your wife does know.

Arthur: I'll give her hell for keeping it from me.

Sister: Why do you think she's kept if from you?

Arthur: 'Cos it's too painful to talk about.

Tears again

Sister: Yes, because she loves you so much. You've both known for a long time, but both in your own way have been trying to protect each other.

Arthur: They don't make women like my wife any more. I'll have to get home to get my affairs sorted out, but she'll be well provided for.

Sister: She's lucky to have a husband like you.

Arthur: We've been married for thirty-eight years. We've had our ups and downs, but I've never even looked at another woman.

Sister: Do you think you will be able to share this with her? After thirty-eight years of never keeping secrets from one another, it seems sad to both go through this alone. I'm sure it would be a bit easier to face if you could face it together.

Arthur: I'll have to think about it. I've got a lot of thinking to do. I'm sorry I've got so emotional. I've never been like this in my life before and I've got you upset too, I can see.

Sister: I feel very proud that you've trusted me enough to let me share it with you a bit.

Arthur: Well, thank you for being so straight with me. That's what I really like about you. Shall I take those bloody pain-killers now, before I go and ring the wife?

That evening Arthur had a completely open conversation with his wife and son. The following week he went home for a few hours and put his affairs in order, explaining all his financial documents to his son. He lived for another five weeks, during which he never once mentioned his imminent death again. He did make one indirect reference to his conversation with the nursing sister, however. He overheard her telephoning some relatives to inform them of a sudden deterioration in a patient's condition. Afterwards, he said to her, 'That's what I like about you, you're honest, bloody honest, even when it's hard'.

During the weeks between the conversation and his death, Arthur relaxed visibly. His medication was eventually halved and he became fully alert and lucid again, but there was no increase in the pain.

CONSPIRACIES OF SILENCE (MUTUAL PRETENCE)

Many dying patients choose not to share their knowledge and feelings with the people closest to them. This is partly in an attempt to protect them from the pain that such a sharing would cause, but also to protect themselves from the pain of facing up to the whole truth. The friends or relatives are frequently doing exactly the same. Sometimes, this conspiracy of silence contains an element of self-pretence, kidding oneself that the partner does not know the true facts; at other times, both partners acknowledge to themselves that the other one knows, but cannot bear to share it. As the weeks pass by and the imminence of death becomes apparent, one or both partners often start to regret this lack of sharing. Many married couples claim never to have kept a single secret from each other in the past and hate the thought of their final parting being marred by this deceit. Others feel they simply cannot cope with their overwhelming fears of death or bereavement without their partner's support. Whatever the reason, patients and relatives sometimes ask members of the nursing staff for help to break through this conspiracy, as they no longer have the strength to do it alone.

Often, very little is required from the person whose help is sought. An interview may be arranged with both partners together. One possible opening could be, 'I know how worried you've both been about Kath's illness, and you've both told me how much you want to talk together about it, but how hard it is to broach the subject. Well, I can understand why that is, because neither of you can bear to see the other hurt and upset. But I know that there are lots of things you really want to say to each other. Tom can't bear to see you so ill Kath, without being able to share your fears and feeling as close to you as he's always been. And Kath can't bear to see you contemplating the future alone Tom, without being able to share your grief and help you make some preparation. I suppose the thing that has stopped you both from talking openly together, because it is just too frightening, is the knowledge that Kath is dying and may not live for very much longer now'.

It is important that the word 'death' or 'dying' is used, so that neither the patient nor the relative is left to introduce the most painful word. Without this, progress in relating to one another may not occur. As soon as a rapport is initiated or, as frequently happens, the tears begin to flow, it is usually time for the mediator to leave the room, allowing the couple the privacy to comfort each other. This intervention may seem a small service, but the difference which is made by reopening such vital channels of communication must be colossal, judging by the amount of gratitude which one receives for helping in such cases.

NON-VERBAL COMMUNICATION

No form of communication is more valuable in terminal care than the non-verbal. Patients who have previously been repulsed by, and afraid of, ill people will be greatly reassured by physical contact, such as the doctor who shakes the patient by the hand in a very positive way on each meeting and parting, the nurse or friend who reaches out and holds a hand, particularly when painful thoughts are being shared. Although most patients experiencing acute grief or fear will long for someone to hold them close, some would be further distressed by such intimacy; great sensitivity is needed.

It has already been mentioned how one's manner can indicate the willingness or lack of it to enter into the patient's world of fear. Those who are afraid or unwilling to share the burden need not worry. It takes great effort to win a patient's trust and he will certainly not thrust his confidence on anyone whose manner is saying, 'I'm afraid of you' or 'Do cheer up and talk about jolly things'.

The manner in which we handle a grossly weak or paralysed patient can make him feel cherished and respected, simply by washing or moving him in a gentle, unhurried way. Sadly, it is equally easy to make him feel like an inanimate object by rough, hurried and careless handling. Many of the kindest nurses would be horrified if they could watch themselves manhandling their patients in the way that they do. Busyness has a lot to answer for.

When a patient or relative asks a difficult question, one which may have a painful answer, he will be watching the face of the person he asks before the answer comes. Will he see the averted eyes, the embarrassment, the anxiety, or will eye-to-eye contact be maintained, assuring him of an honest answer? Verbal communication can say what we want it to say, not necessarily the truth or what we feel. Non-verbal communication reveals our true feelings and the vulnerability of someone who is dying makes him especially sensitive to this.

COMMUNICATION WITH AN UNCONSCIOUS PATIENT

When a patient has lost consciousness, particularly while the level is still light, he may continue to be aware of sound and touch, plus the other senses to a lesser degree. Even when deeply unconscious, it would appear that there is sometimes an awareness of the presence of other people. This is often demonstrated by the patient who seems distressed and restless when left alone, but who becomes immediately peaceful when someone is sitting with him. It is vital, therefore, to handle him as gently, carefully and in as unhurried a way as the conscious patient. Clear explanations should be given before undertaking any procedures such as catheterisation, turning or the giving of injections. Reassurances that pain will be kept under control and information about who is in the room, which visitor has arrived, or what time of day it is, will greatly increase the patient's peace of mind. Physical contact, such as stroking the unconscious person's head or holding his hand, is comforting to both the patient and their loved one. Many people who have cared for someone throughout an illness become distanced once the patient loses consciousness. This is partly due to fear, and partly due to their lack of knowledge about the level of awareness which may be retained when someone is only lightly unconscious.

Relatives will need a great deal of information, support and understanding from the nurses involved to enable them to continue to participate in the care, and they will need to see the example of someone more experienced talking to the patient and holding his hand before they will have the confidence to do likewise. Many painful feelings of uselessness and guilt can be avoided by enabling the spouse, daughter or friend to continue to care for their loved one and stay close to him, even after he has lost consciousness. Too many people are left to their own devices at this stage. Often they are actively encouraged to withdraw and are then left to wander round in a state of inertia for days on end.

COUNSELLING

Everyone involved in the care of the dying will need to develop their own counselling skills. These will be used primarily in the support of patients and their families, but they may also be helpful in meeting the needs of colleagues.

The term 'counselling' has come into vogue with a vengeance in the past ten years or so, a period during which the understanding of psychology by the lay public has escalated and the importance of inter-personal relationships has become widely recognised. The ever increasing quantity of literature on the subject, and the wide variety of training courses available, have led many nurses to envisage counselling as a totally new and alien art, in which they feel unskilled, untrained and inadequate. However, the truth is that counselling has always been a major part of the nurse's role. The discovery and recognition of the significance of counselling should not be seen as a threat to the role of the nurse. Any increase in organised forms of caring within society should be welcomed and encouraged, since this is the very essence of nursing. The introduction of counselling to the nursing curriculum is proving to be of great value, although it is likely that learning by example, in the wards, will continue to be the mode of teaching which carries greatest impact.

COUNSELLING COURSES

An increasing number of nurses are making use of the specific courses on counselling which are available to them. These are usually part-time, multi-disciplinary courses, often run by the local education authority, charitable bodies such as 'Cruse' or the 'Institute of Group Analysis', but the Royal College of Nursing also runs courses which are purely for nurses. The courses come in all shapes and sizes, but most contain a large experiential element, aimed at increasing the student's level of self-awareness. They are, therefore, potentially as painful as they are rewarding. Some also include relationship studies, which enable the students to bring work situations to the course for analysis, role-playing, support and often guidance for the future. The final element of the typical counselling course, and the one always given least emphasis, is the teaching of theories and techniques. Some of this is based on the traditional theories of psychology, psychotherapy and psychoanalysis, but grounding may also be given in some of the more recently developed theories of counselling, such as the Rogerian method, developed by Carl Rogers, re-evaluation counselling, developed by Harvey Jackins, and transactional analysis, developed by Eric Berne. These theories all tend to be more circumscribed and dogmatic than the traditional approach. Counselling courses are generally unstructured, with the tutors taking a non-directive approach. This method of teaching and learning is very different from that to which many nurses are accustomed. Feelings of insecurity and frustration at not being 'taught anything' are common.

THE AIMS OF COUNSELLING

The type of counselling which this form of training is geared to is, basically, therapeutic communication. This is usually between two people, the counsellor and the client, though it can also be practised in a group setting. The client is any person seeking help with a psychological or emotional problem. It is important to remember that they are not normally psychiatrically ill. They are usually people who are psychologically healthy, but who are seeking help to cope with the normal pains of living. The counsellor is any person offering to meet this need. The skill of the latter may be the result of a full, professional training in psychiatry, psychotherapy or psychoanalysis, or it may be the most humble expertise of one who has learned 'on the job', with the help of part-time courses such as those described above. The aim of counselling is to relate and respond to the client in such a way that he is helped to explore his own thoughts, feelings and behaviour, thereby increasing his understanding of himself and his situation. The client is often able to function more effectively with this increased clarity and objectivity, and, as a result, to feel more at peace with himself and the world.

THE PRACTICE OF COUNSELLING

If a patient or relative is found in a state of obvious distress, the nurse's priorities should be so ordered that she will, if at all possible, immediately delegate her next hour's responsibilities, remembering that, like everyone else, she is not indispensable. She will then take the distressed person into a private place, leaving a firm request for no interruptions or telephone calls. Once privacy and peace have been established, the counsellor will seat herself close to the client, preferably in an easy chair, or on the edge of the bed if the patient is not able to get up, but never behind a desk.

The confidentiality with which any exchange of information will be treated by the counsellor may seem too obvious to be worth mentioning. However, for the benefit of those clients less familiar with the ethics of counselling, it is important that this should be made quite clear.

An atmosphere of great safety must be created for any useful sharing to be possible. This is achieved by what the counsellor says and by her manner, but most of all by her own feelings, which will communicate themselves to the client. The counsellor will need to initiate the conversation, taking full responsibility for establishing a rapport. The distressed and vulnerable client cannot be expected to meet her half-way, as is the case with most inter-personal relationships. The three factors which the counsellor needs to convey to the client, above all else, are respect, empathy and acceptance, sometimes described in counselling jargon as 'unconditional positive regard'.

Within this environment the client will be able to work on his feelings, be they grief, fear, anger, frustration or despair. This may be done by talking through the events which have given rise to the distress, by working out connections with previous experiences which may have increased the present response, and also by emotional discharge in forms such as tears, trembling, or rage. The counsellor's role is to listen attentively to what is being said, encouraging and supporting the client to reach his own increased understanding of himself and his problems, reaching his own conclusions and making his own decisions for the future. The client will require encouragement to release emotion, not soothing in order to subdue the outburst. This can only be achieved if the counsellor remains unaffected, displaying neither shock nor distress, accepting the feelings with no hint of judgement. Physical contact may increase the necessary safety but, in some people, the reverse occurs, and the tears and rage are suppressed.

The counsellor will observe all non-verbal forms of communication, including posture, tone of voice, hand movements, facial expressions and general attitude, often learning far more from these, and from what the client omits to say, than from the spoken word. It is important not to interrupt the flow of thoughts and not to fill up periods of silence, since these are essential thinking time. However, sometimes it will be helpful for the counsellor to reflect back, in her own words, what she has heard the client saying, checking the accuracy of her interpretation. She may also recount some of the feelings she has observed the client expressing non-verbally, of which the latter may be quite unaware. This technique will encourage the client to clarify his thinking further, as he corrects any misinterpretations.

Amidst the hurly-burly of everyday life, few people ever receive this quality of attention for a sustained period. During normal conversation, the participants are often more concerned with getting their next contribution in than with hearing what the other person is saying. But this sustained, uncritical attention is essential for emotional health. Consequently, those new to counselling are often surprised by the depth of response which their attitude and attention unleash.

More experienced and knowledgeable counsellors may use a far more directive approach. They may encourage the client to explore the painful areas he seems to be avoiding, or they may confront his defence mechanisms, such as denial, repression or projection. Some will use 'free association', which they then interpret, and they may also offer interpretations of dreams, fantasies and drawings, as well as of the thinking which the client shares during the session. All experienced counsellors use the relationship which develops between themselves and the client as a therapeutic tool, since this will not only highlight relationship difficulties, but will also provide the opportunity to work on them. (Not all of the distress experienced by dying patients and their families is directly concerned with illness and death; a great deal of it is to do with relationship difficulties.) These techniques would only be embarked upon by those with psychotherapeutic or psychoanalytical skills, however, since they can be harmful if used by those with insufficient expertise. The client, stripped of his defences, can become extremely vulnerable.

It is important that the counsellor stays close to the client, even when she finds that she is experiencing some of his pain herself. But these feelings should not be expressed or acted upon at the time. Any such demonstration of the nurse's own feelings could inhibit further sharing by the patient or relative. This is not to say that a few tears trickling down the face of someone who is counselling a grieving relative are unacceptable. What is important is that the attention remains one hundred per cent on the patient or relative, and that none is focussed on the nurse's own feelings at the time. To provide effective support, one must be capable of taking a detached and objective view of what is going on. This degree of empathy, combined with detachment and self-control, puts a tremendous strain on the counsellor.

Should the person in the counselling role succumb to a compulsive desire to impose details of her own similar experiences upon the client, or if there is any indication of dwindling interest, the client's ability to share his feelings may once again be inhibited. Counsellors must be willing and able to be temporarily on the giving end of a non-reciprocal relationship. Needless to say, their needs must also be met at a later date, and the imbalance redressed.

The apparent inability to give one-way attention is often due to the arousal of painful feelings, caused by associations or memories of events similar to those being described by the client. To prevent these feelings from blocking any future communication, they will need to be explored, probably with the help of another counsellor. By acknowledging their presence and allowing oneself to re-experience the pain they produce, much of the related distress can often be released, freeing one's future attention for the client.

The high quality attention required from the counsellor demands total commitment. If the counsellor is already drained by the day's work, and the distress is not of an acute nature, it may be better to make an appointment for another day.

Many people who are dying, and many of those close to someone who is dying, will need regular counselling sessions for a very long time. It is, therefore, important for the nurse-counsellor to recognise her limitations in terms of time, as well as expertise, and to be aware of the existence of local counselling services to which clients may need to be referred. Other members of the team, particularly the social worker or psychiatrist, may be more appropriate than the nurse in supporting those with obviously complex and long-term needs. Counselling should never be embarked upon casually. A strong, personal commitment to work with the client is essential. During the terminal stage of a fatal illness, sessions may need to be as often as daily, and total reliability with regard to punctuality and availability for all appointments is extremely important. Consequently, although nurses may do a great deal of spontaneous counselling, particularly when patients or relatives are in acute distress, they are often unable to meet the practical demands of a pre-arranged series of interviews, and will, therefore, have to refer the client to a suitable colleague, usually the medical social worker.

Chapter 5

The Psychological Adaptation to Death

Those approaching death have been described by numerous psychiatrists, physicians and psychologists as passing through a predictable series of classic emotional stages. In reality, these are often difficult to distinguish as they vary enormously in length and intensity from person to person, with a unique mode of presentation for each individual. There is usually a great deal of 'to-ing and fro-ing', progressing from one stage into the next, then regressing into an earlier one again, the stages frequently overlapping one another or being omitted altogether. However, it is useful to have a basic concept of these stages, as a baseline from which to start thinking when faced with the complexity of emotional turmoil, present in most patients when approaching death.

As previously described, the awareness of the possibility of death and, later, its imminence, is not necessarily dependent on a doctor's diagnostic or prognostic revelations. Consequently, the process of adaptation may begin at any time. It could be at an early stage of the disease, when a breast lump is first discovered, for instance, or it may not begin until physical deterioration makes awareness unavoidable.

The stages described vary in number, title and content from author to author, so the account of the eight stages which follows is simply a personal interpretation derived from encounters with dying patients.

SHOCK

Shock can be seen as a protective blanket which is thrown over us whenever our emotions are aroused so violently that we are at risk of being overwhelmed by them. However gradually and sensitively a patient is given information about his illness, he is almost certain to experience waves of shock. They may also be triggered off by the appearance of new symptoms, the discovery of a massive weight loss, another lump, or the sight of blood in the sputum, for example.

Shock can take one of two forms. It may present as panic, with hyperactivity, compulsive talking, insomnia and a general air of agitation. With almost equal frequency it will present as numbness, with apathy, inactivity and an abnormal calm. The blood pressure of those who are numbed or stunned may drop very low, and fainting is not uncommon.

Any of the physical symptoms of acute anxiety may be seen in either form of shock. These include tachycardia, sweating, swings in body temperature, trembling, 'butterflies in the tummy', nausea, anorexia, frequency of micturition and diarrhoea.

DENIAL

Denial can be a most valuable defence mechanism, and it is frequently employed for a variable period of time as the symptoms of shock diminish. The patient avoids any discussion of his diagnosis or prognosis, desperately trying to live a totally normal existence. Even thinking about the possible or imminent death is avoided and hyperactivity is common. Every waking moment is filled with activity so that there is no time for painful thoughts to surface.

When denial is used most forcibly, patients may trek from one doctor to the next in an attempt to procure a different medical opinion. Others will avoid further contact with their doctor, failing to attend every appointment made. When information is imparted in a brusque, blunt manner by a doctor with whom the patient has only a superficial relationship, a prolonged period of denial seems far more common. Ironically, the doctors who perform this most clumsily are often those who care the most, and who are, therefore, most distressed by the task of imparting such news. There is an urgent need for better training in this field.

However openly a patient may have discussed the future on other occasions, periods of denial may still be re-entered, perhaps as the only means of defence, when the full impact of reality seems intolerable. It is only harmful when employed continuously, causing the painful feelings about dying to be suppressed. When denial is used intermittently, those supporting the patient need to be extra sensitive to his frame of mind, permitting denial one moment and supporting him to deal with his awareness of the truth the next. The sharing of very real grief, such as that felt about not seeing a young family grow up, may follow hot on the heels of conversations like, 'When I'm better and this is all behind me, we're going to buy a house in Spain'.

Fortunately, most people find at least one person with whom they feel sufficiently safe to be able to admit to their awareness of the true situation, even if they are denying it with everyone else. It may not be a close relative or friend, since this would inevitably entail coping with the exposure of their grief also, but it may well be the district nurse, the home help, or an understanding neighbour whom they choose.

If health visitors are informed by their general practitioners whenever a patient has been confronted with a fatal diagnosis, they can play an important role. They will not only be able to clarify, repeat and elaborate on the information given by the doctor, but they will be able to provide the high quality of attention needed by the patient to help him come to terms with its implications for the future.

It is almost never appropriate to try and force a person who is denying the truth to acknowledge it. Those who seem to be permanently in this stage have often avoided or denied all painful experiences throughout their lives, and are unlikely to be able to change at this time. However, denial in a dying person will often involve the suppression of very powerful emotions, such as fear, anger and grief. Very occasionally, this will cause the patient to suffer so greatly that confrontation with the truth is the kindest approach. Severe anxiety and frequent nightmares are sometimes indicators that this is the case.

The two accounts which follow are both examples of patients who used denial almost continuously.

Tim

Tim was fifty-one years old, a divorcee and the father of a thirteen-year-old daughter and a sixteen-year-old son, both of whom were still at school. Having been left by his wife two years previously, Tim had gained custody of the children, who had seen their mother only once during the eighteen months since the divorce.

Tim's diagnosis was a rapidly growing oat cell carcinoma of the right bronchus. He had been given both radiotherapy and a long course of chemotherapy. The time had come to discontinue the latter, as it was proving ineffective and its side-effects were so harmful and unpleasant. No other form of palliative treatment was available and Tim was obviously in the terminal stages of his illness. He was admitted to hospital at this time because of severe dyspnoea and increasing weakness.

It was ascertained from the family doctor and the oncologist that Tim had never asked about his diagnosis. He had in fact made it impossible for either of them to tell him by always changing the subject, or rushing off whenever the matter was raised. The children apparently knew nothing about their father's condition either, although, according to their teachers, they were showing considerable signs of stress at school.

It was obviously quite out of the question to leave the children unprepared for their father's death and to have made no plans for their future care.

After a great deal of thought, discussion and a case conference, it was decided that Tim should be told about his diagnosis and the brevity of his prognosis, so that he could decide who should tell the children and be involved in supporting them and planning for their future.

After two weeks in hospital, Tim was considerably weaker. He was extremely anxious. His pupils were widely dilated, he sweated profusely and was always active, however tired, usually turning out his bedside locker. He slept for short periods only during the night, pacing around the unit when awake. In his relationships with the staff he always managed to be cheery and jovial, and all attempts to encourage him to talk realistically about his situation were rebuffed.

The day after the case conference, Tim asked one of the sisters which day his chemotherapy would be given that week. She repeated the information that had already been given by the doctor, that the treatment was being discontinued. He then asked if the course had been completed and said it had not done much good. The sister explained exactly why it had been discontinued. Tim said nothing, but looked very frightened. She then asked him if he understood what was wrong with him and if the children knew how ill he was. He looked like a trapped animal as he revealed his knowledge of his diagnosis and asked if he had any hope of pulling through. He said that the children did not know, and although he did not want to see his wife, he wanted her to be informed of his diagnosis so that she could tell them. He also made it quite clear that he thought the children would want to be with their mother after his death, and that she should come and be with them meanwhile.

At the end of a very lengthy interview, Tim asked for the curtains to be pulled around his bed. He wept for nearly two hours, staunchly refusing to allow anyone to sit with him.

The next day he told the sister very bitterly that she should never have told him that he was dying, and that no one had the right to tell anyone that kind of thing. Although she had given no time limit to his life expectation and had been as gentle as she was able, he was seething with anger and resentment. His son visited alone that afternoon and Tim decided to tell him the score himself. They cried together, holding hands for a long time.

That evening Tim quite clearly turned his face to the wall. He took to his bed and buried his face under the bedclothes, refusing to eat, drink or communicate. Within twenty-four hours he was extremely drowsy and doubly incontinent. In forty-eight hours he was unconscious and two days later he died.

Ruth

Ruth was the forty-year-old mother of a fourteen-year-old daughter and a sixteen-year-old son. Her husband had worked his way up from the shop floor to become a company director. They seemed a very happy and united family. Ruth had been a beautician before her marriage and had, of late, done a lot of voluntary beauty work in several old people's homes and a unit for the young disabled.

The original diagnosis was breast cancer, but since a mastectomy two and half years earlier the disease had spread to the lymph nodes, brain and ribs. Oncological treatments had been given one after the other, despite which the tumour had recurred at the mastectomy site and in the other breast, and the whole area was fungating. When treatment was under way Ruth seemed cheerful and well able to cope, but when nothing was being done or planned she would get very agitated and anxious. On several of these occasions, she referred herself to other consultants privately for second opinions.

During her many admissions for pain control in the later stages of her illness, she was physically very disfigured. The dexamethasone for her cerebral metastases had caused her to become grossly overweight and cushinoid. The breast fungation was enormous and extremely unsightly, chemotherapy had caused her to lose all her hair, and lymphatic obstruction had caused her left arm to be about double its normal size. In addition, Ruth was dyspnoeic on minimal exertion, and yet her will to live and her determination to beat the disease were as strong as they had ever been.

Hyperactivity and tremendous bravado were Ruth's hallmarks. Her chatter and laughter could be heard all over the unit and examples of her wide variety of handicrafts were strewn everywhere. Her day was geared from one visitor to the next. She acknowledged openly her dependence on company and demanded that the staff spent time with her whenever she was on her own. As her condition worsened, she became even more afraid of being alone. She would not go into her bedroom from the time she got up in the morning until her night sedatives were actually taking effect.

The time eventually came when Ruth's family felt that they could no longer manage to care for her at home, even intermittently. The discharge and stench from the breast lesion, the increasing physical instability from the cerebral tumours, plus her behaviour, which was by now quite hysterical at times, were too much for them to cope with.

Several times a day, she would demand to know when she would be well enough to go home. Several times a day, she would plead with one member of staff after another to share her belief that she was going to get well again and live. Her anger with those who felt unable to give empty reassurances knew no bounds. She would say over and over again that she could not possibly die, that she must get better, that she would get better, and why did the staff not believe her, they must believe her. Her bargaining with God was very evident. She not only persuaded her daughter to begin confirmation classes but was confirmed herself. Her attendance at services soon ceased however, as her condition continued to deteriorate.

As her death became imminent, Ruth's husband tried to discuss with her how he should prepare the children. This was the last straw. Even her husband was betraying her and losing faith in her recovery. She screamed at him in a wild frenzy for ten minutes or more, ending in desperate sobs, but she would not allow him to comfort her. This was the first time that she had cried since her mastectomy. Her frequent outbursts of laughter had so often seemed void of all happiness, serving merely as a means of quelling the tears she so badly needed to shed.

Ruth died very angry. She felt as though the truth she had refused to accept had been thrust upon her. Had the staff gone along with her attempt at self-deceit, it is doubtful whether she would have fared any better, for she would have known deep down that her condition was deteriorating daily and would have felt unable to trust them. She tried desperately to fight the drowsiness as she began to lose consciousness and, even when unconscious, she was excessively restless, as though fighting right to the bitter end.

BARGAINING

This stage involves the negotiation of an agreement with God, fate, or whatever one happens to call the ultimate power. Although far less likely to occur in a convinced atheist, it is not unknown. A pledge is made by the dying person to become less selfish, to do some altruistic deed, to attend church regularly, or to accept a certain degree of disablement and pain without complaint. In return, he demands longevity.

Although only a small number of people admit to doing this with any great sincerity, many dying patients, particularly the younger ones, admit to having caught themselves conjuring up such agreements, if only in a fairly sceptical or light-hearted manner. This may well be due to embarrassment or fear of being ridiculed.

In some cases, the bargain or agreement is made by the patient with himself. Although accepting that the medical world cannot provide a cure, he determines to beat the disease by 'mind over matter'. Goals may be set, such as the birth of a grandchild, or Christmas. The patient promises himself that he will keep going until the goal is reached, come what may. Of course the mental attitude can affect the prognosis, and sadly, many patients with this kind of determination struggle on long after all quality of life appears to have been lost.

ANGER

In an age when longevity is regarded as everyone's birthright, and automation has so freed us from the rigorous labours of our ancestors, that a high level of introspection and egocentricity are the norm, anger at one's life being extinguished prematurely can be colossal. For most people this is the most difficult emotion to discharge, as any angry, aggressive outburst carries with it the danger of alienation and isolation from those whose support is so vital. It is, therefore, the emotion most often suppressed, and consequently one of those most likely to exacerbate physical pain.

Anger is almost always displaced onto those people with whom the patient feels safest and by whom they feel most loved and respected. However, it is sometimes displaced onto the medical staff who have failed to effect a cure. Although nursing staff may also be the target for anger, they usually escape this. Most patients feel a little too dependent on their nurses, in addition to which it is far safer to display anger towards someone who spends ten minutes a day with you than someone who is around for eight or ten hours.

Alternatively, the anger may be directed at God. This seems to be the most rational target for the anger of anyone who believes in an omnipotent God. Anxious clergymen, trying to quell any admission of this feeling, may need encouragement to allow patients to express their anger. It is sometimes useful to ask them why they think they need to jump to God's defence. Are they saying that God cannot, or will not, cope with anger? It may be easier to demonstrate the harm that this anger can do when aimed at relatives already debilitated by grief, or to the patient himself when it is suppressed.

Anger often gives rise to questions such as 'Why me?', or 'I've always tried to be a good husband and father – where did I go wrong?'. The nurse's first response is almost always to try and find an answer, but it soon becomes clear that answers are not what the patient needs. She has to learn to listen to these questions and to feel the underlying anger, without defending herself with words. By showing that she too has no answers, and that she can empathise with his feelings, the patient may feel safe enough to acknowledge and reveal a bit more of his anger.

It is far harder to be on the receiving end of a patient's anger than to share his grief or despair. Many relatives will have been making the most enormous sacrifices in order to give their loved one the very best care possible, and will be hurt and baffled by the anger which is displaced onto them. They will need a great deal of help, not only to understand why they have been chosen as the target for the anger, which seems so unjustified, but also to deal with their own hurt feelings. Only when this type of support is provided will the relative be able to remain close and loving to the patient, refraining from retaliation or withdrawal. Doctors and nurses will need similar help if they are the focus upon which the anger is directed.

The following case study relates to a young woman who showed no sign of anger. But could anyone of her age really accept that they were dying without experiencing any anger at all?

Anne

Anne was a twenty-eight-year-old social worker. She was single, but had strong relationships with her family and some very close friends. She had been diagnosed as having Hodgkin's disease for over five years. During that time she had led a very full life, clinging onto the possibility of a cure, but gradually realising that this was not to be. By the time she was admitted to hospital for terminal care she was well aware that she was dying. Her overriding symptom at this time was intolerable, intractable pain. Every type of drug and pain-relieving procedure had failed, and only by prescribing diamorphine at the rate of 120mg subcutaneously every three hours was it possible to achieve any relief.

Anne was a very gentle, caring person. Even though she was so ill, she was always thoughtful and courteous. Being a social worker she had access to a college library, from which she had borrowed every book to be found on the subject of Hodgkin's disease and those about dying. She talked very openly and unemotionally about her imminent death. She claimed to feel no great anguish about it, just a little sadness over those she was leaving behind, whilst her main feeling was one of acceptance of the goodness and timeliness of her death. She was an ardent naturalist and intellectually accepted her death as a very natural and good part of her life cycle.

As there was no physical explanation for pain of this severity, it can only be supposed that it may have been due to a great deal of suppressed fear and anger. It was as though her emotional reaction to death had been unable to live up to the expectations of her sophisticated intellectual reaction. But like all strong emotion which is suppressed, it was certain to find some means of expressing itself.

This can only be a supposition, for any attempts to facilitate the expression of fear and anger were forestalled by a rapid physical deterioration. Although somewhat euphoric as a result of the huge doses of diamorphine, at least Anne's last days were virtually pain-free.

DEPRESSION

All the stages and emotions so far described have demanded a great deal of effort and energy, but as anger subsides and denial and bargaining break down, many patients seem too weary to go on fighting, and despair and depression creep in. They are now consciously aware of their impending death.

There is so much to feel depressed about. Some of the more likely causes are the pain of anticipated loss, which will embrace everybody and everything that has ever been valued, sadness over all those things never to be achieved, guilt and regret about pain caused to others during one's life, and the loss of safety as one approaches an unfamiliar void.

At this time, the will to go on living whatever time is left appears to have been sapped. Insomnia and anorexia, in addition to the weakness caused by the disease, leave the patient weary of life. Tears flow most readily now and these can only hasten the resolution of the depression. The nurse's role is to permit and encourage the sharing of distressing thoughts and feelings, remembering that it is never possible or appropriate to try to cheer a depressed person up. Sadly, many patients remain in this state of depression until they die. A few will take their own lives, feeling that life of this quality, with a death-sentence hanging over them, is intolerable.

The following account shows how some of the deepest depression seen in those who are dying is experienced by those who have least to lose.

Ada

Ada was fifty-eight years old when she developed motor neurone disease. Her father had died when she was a child, but she had continued to live with her mother and brother until nine years ago, when first her brother, and soon after, her mother, had died. She was a shy, withdrawn person who had no friends or relations, and she led a solitary, secluded life. She was employed as a book-keeper at a small tailor's shop.

Twelve months after the diagnosis was made, Ada had to give up her job, because she no longer had the muscle-power in her arms to write or type for more than a few minutes at a time. Six months later, she was not even able to wash or feed herself and was admitted to a hospice.

It took a long time to overcome her barriers of reserve, but the nurses were careful not to hurry her or to force their attentions upon her. Ada's speech was difficult to understand and this undermined her confidence still further. Other patients and their visitors, seeing how isolated she was, frequently gave her small gifts of fruit or sweets and tried to include her in their conversations. Unfortunately, her shyness made her seem very ungracious, so they usually gave up, feeling rebuffed, after a few attempts.

When feeding Ada, the nurses made a point of talking very little, partly because it was necessary to concentrate hard in order to avoid making her choke, and partly because it was impossible for her to respond when eating. When she was having her daily bath, however, they would talk quietly to her, avoiding intimate or threatening subjects. Eventually, after four or five weeks in the hospice, she began to use the privacy and safety of bath-time to unburden some of her sadness.

The thought which seemed to cause Ada the most pain, and the one she repeated and wept over almost every day, was that her life held no value. She felt that she had contributed nothing at all to society and that her death would have no meaning for anyone. She felt that she would leave no gap anywhere and that all memory of her existence would fade in a matter of weeks.

Although she had virtually no visitors, Ada refused all forms of diversional therapy which were offered to her. She did not read, listen to the radio or television, do any form of handcraft or join in any social activities which took place in the hospice day unit. She refused the offer of a volunteer to become her regular visitor, and she refused the offers of two members of the nursing staff to take her out for a drive. Most days she would spend her time lying on the bed with her eyes closed.

Ada was particularly difficult to nurse because, unlike most dying patients who move in and out of periods of sadness, she appeared to be depressed all of the time. Whenever she did converse openly, she always expressed bitterness about the mode of her dying and the length of time it was taking. She also expressed regret that she had not taken an overdose at the outset of the illness, when she was still able to do so, although she never referred to the possibility of euthanasia.

A course of antidepressant drugs was commenced with Ada's consent, but these had to be discontinued because of respiratory difficulties. As the disease had begun in the upper motor neurones, she was already finding breathing a problem, without any further depression of the respiratory centre.

It can only be hoped that the efforts made in trying to care for Ada made some impression, however slight, on her unhappiness. She died after four and a half months in the unit and her death seemed to be very peaceful.

FEAR

Even if no other emotion is evident, fear is the one that few dying patients succeed in concealing. Having once realised that death is imminent, fear of the mode of dying and of the life (or lack of it) to come, is universal. Waves of fear come sweeping over with many of the physical components of acute anxiety, caused by the stimulation of the sympathetic nervous system and the inhibition of the parasympathetic. The most common symptoms are increased heart and respiratory rates, increased muscle tension, nausea due to relaxation of intestinal muscle, a dry mouth due to suppression of salivary production and a cold, clammy feeling due to increased sweating and constriction of peripheral blood vessels. These feelings of overwhelming fear are not experienced continuously, however. The experience of dying has been likened to war – five per cent terror and and ninety-five per cent hanging around waiting.

Like any other fear, the fear of dying is likely to be worse at night when feelings of isolation are heightened and there is no other stimulus to help balance out the feelings. The darkness seems to magnify fear a hundredfold. In the familiarity of one's own home, especially if there is someone sleeping beside you, the fear may not be quite so intense and it is certainly easier to ask for the comfort and support required. In hospital, nurses on night-duty need to be especially observant, recognising fear when they see it and demonstrating great compassion. Unlimited cups of tea are so often served up to the restless patient, merely keeping him on the trot to the lavatory all night, when what is really needed is a little time and attention for the sharing of fears. Male patients are often reluctant to admit that they are afraid, feeling that it is unmanly and a sign of weakness. However, far greater frankness and intimacy often seem possible in the small hours of the night than ever occurs in the light of day.

It has often been claimed that those with a firm faith, whatever their religion, and those quite certain of their atheism, have the least fear of death, whilst the 'unsures' suffer the most. This does not always seem to be the case, however. Many committed Christians obtain great comfort from their expectation of the life hereafter, but it is also clear that many others experience a great exacerbation of their fears if their faith includes the less fashionable notions of 'a Day of Judgement' and punishment by 'hell, fire and damnation'. They seem like two entirely opposite faiths, one in a God of love and forgiveness and the other in a God of power and punishment. However, this is a naive interpretation, for it is perfectly feasible to fear a God of love. When approaching death, the thought of seeing one's own inadequacies compared with pure love must be a daunting prospect. A priest whose faith does not encompass the fear of punishment after death may find it difficult to comfort a patient experiencing this, for a lifetime of fear is not easily erased.

Many believers seem too ashamed to acknowledge their fears about death and dying, imagining that this would constitute a denial of their faith. Once again, it may fall to the priest to give permission and encouragement to express these feelings.

REGRESSION

Although usually a symptom of depression, regression is further encouraged by the physical loss of independence in the terminally ill. Incontinence, gross weakness, confusional states and drowsiness necessitate the provision of personal care normally reserved for children. The emotionally regressive patient can become childlike, with spouse and nurse taking on the parental role. It is not easy to perform tasks of basic hygiene, such as bathing, toileting and dressing for another adult, while maintaining a peer relationship. Regression, however, can only lead to further demoralisation through loss of dignity and self-respect.

Relatives and friends find it especially difficult to watch a weak patient laboriously performing some minor task which they themselves could do in a matter of seconds. The nursing staff should set an example for them by encouraging patients to maintain the maximum amount of independence possible, however slowly or laboriously they perform the simplest of tasks, such as cleaning their own teeth or getting dressed. Although a great deal of effort may be required from the patient, the satisfaction which can be derived from these achievements should not be underestimated.

Both medical and nursing staff have a responsibility to ensure that patients are sufficiently well informed about their condition, and the treatment options available, that they can be involved in all decisions made about their own medical management. Many patients will be reluctant to be involved, but collusion in this matter by the medical staff will only help to increase the degree of dependency and regression and the consequent demoralisation.

Regression is a defence mechanism, and the following account demonstrates this clearly. It is used here to avoid the grief which seemed inevitable to a mature adult, Walter.

Walter

Walter was a fifty-eight-year-old Polish Jew, though not a practising one, married to an English wife. They had no children. Three years previously, he had had a large area of bowel resected because of a squamous cell carcinoma. An end-to-end anastamosis had been performed. The tumour had recently recurred causing a subacute bowel obstruction, but further surgery was considered to be meddlesome, due to the extent of the liver metastases.

The main reasons that necessitated Walter's admission to hospital were the changes in his personality and his wife's need for a period of respite. He had always been a fastidious, pedantic person, but these facets of his personality were now so exaggerated that they had become intolerable for his wife to contend with, living alone with him, twenty-four hours a day.

Walter had his own company, manufacturing toys. His weakness and extreme anxiety had rendered him incapable of performing his very responsible job any longer, but despite encouragement from his colleagues, his secretary and his wife to hand over the reins for a while, he was still attempting to run the business from his bed. Admitting Walter to hospital greatly heightened his level of anxiety, as a result of which he became increasingly confused and quite unfit to be conducting business affairs. However, as if to prove that he was well, he would frantically write letters, read papers, and make non-stop telephone calls. As time passed, the nonsensical nature of his letters and telephone calls became increasingly apparent and his power to authorise payments and orders had to be legally invalidated for a while.

Walter continued to talk compulsively to anyone who would listen, linking one topic to the next with such speed that it was extremely difficult to escape from him without being rude. He was obsessional about the arrangement of his possessions and papers around his bed, constantly rearranging them, moving things back and forth half an inch until they were just right. His daily ablutions had to follow a very precise pattern and time schedule, and any attempt to fall out of line by the staff would evoke great anger.

He was obviously having extremely frightening nightmares; his sleep was restless and he would cry out in great anguish. On waking he would be flushed and sweating, with a rapid pulse. He was unwilling to share these dreams for several days.

Walter had never asked about his prognosis, but he knew that his original operation was for cancer of the bowel. He left all the open-ended questions like 'You must be feeling pretty worried about yourself . . .' which were offered to him, exactly where they were. However, one night his repeated crying out in his sleep became so disturbing for the other patients that he had to be moved into a single room. At this moment, Walter's defences started to drop for the first time, and in the anonymity of the night he was able to reveal the content of his recurring dreams. They were all based on his memories of war-time experiences, of friends killed alongside him in battle and of his persecution in a prisoner-of-war camp. He said he had had these nightmares intermittently ever since the war, but never to the extent that he was having them now. When questioned about why he thought he might be having them so much more frequently now, he shrugged it off. Within a few days Walter was able to volunteer the possible link between his dreams and his fear of dying.

Almost immediately following this discussion, Walter's behaviour underwent an enormous change. He gave up his pretence of running the company, stopped talking nearly so fast and compulsively, and regressed into a childlike state of dependency. He would take no responsibility for his own personal hygiene, for deciding what to wear or for dressing himself. He would even try to get his wife or the nurses to feed him. Discussion about the possibility of sending him home again provoked something very like a two-year-old's temper tantrum. Not getting his favourite nurse to bath him would get a similar response.

Unfortunately, he never did get home again as he developed a total bowel obstruction. Electrolyte imbalance induced drowsiness and confusion, with a return of all the previous agitation and restlessness. Objects and voices were continually misperceived and misinterpreted, and he would talk to himself in a rambling, incoherent manner. The mental pain he suffered during his time in hospital was minimised by the use of drugs and by the constant care and support of his wife, his doctors and the nursing staff, but it was not possible to relieve it completely.

RESIGNATION

Much has been written about the glorious state of acceptance seen in people who are soon to die. This is, however, a great deal less common than some people would have us believe, and a state of peaceful resignation, accepting what you cannot change, is far more likely to occur. There should be no shame in dying mystified and angry at the painful and premature curtailment of one's life, especially when no faith is aspired to. Those caring for the dying should be wary of the temptation to judge the quality of a death by the patient's degree of acceptance, instead of seeing it in context as a natural consequence of the way he has conducted the rest of his life. Working with dying patients can be very humbling, especially with those who have learned the great art of living one day at a time, determined to live life to the full for as long as they are able to. One frequently experiences such great courage, the strength of which leads many of them, even the parent leaving a young family behind, to say 'If it's got to happen to someone, why not me?'.

Sadly, some patients never reach a stage of peace at all, but remain angry, denying and fighting until they die. Some grow increasingly distressed, making life almost unbearable for their families and those caring for them. This state is best described as one of 'reject and rage'.

Everyone is likely to have some fear of the process of dying, but many will welcome death itself. This group contains those whom the ravages of illness have drained of all will to go on living, the elderly who have grown weary of life, those with exceptional faith, and those whose lives have been so miserable and impoverished, for whatever reason, that death represents an end to their suffering.

As death approaches, many patients seem to enter a twilight state, somewhere between life and death. There is a desire to withdraw from communication, even with loved ones, and any disturbance caused when performing essential nursing care is greatly resented. This may be a defence mechanism, a way of avoiding the pain of parting, but it seems much more concerned with preparing for death. Although conscious, the patient keeps his eyes closed almost all the time and refuses to eat or drink. This is usually a peaceful time and the transition into unconsciousness is often imperceptible. Relatives may feel hurt and rejected, and will need a great deal of support to understand and cope with the situation. They may feel angry with the patient, sensing that he has given up the fight to go on living.

The last two case studies speak for themselves.

Thomas

Thomas was a bachelor of eighty-nine who had worked all his life as a farm labourer. He had been dying slowly for over a year from cirrhosis of the liver, due to a lifetime's excessive intake of alcohol. He was admitted to hospital when no longer able to look after himself, as his only living relative was a brother, almost as old and frail as himself.

He settled into his new environment very quickly, thoroughly enjoying the warmth, the food and his evening beer. Sharing a room with two other smokers, he was also able to enjoy his old pipe without disturbing anyone.

His main symptoms were discomfort, caused by ascites, and weakness, largely caused by anaemia. He had oesophageal varices and haemorrhoids which had bled intermittently for many years, but fortunately this was minimal during his last weeks of life. Apart from trips to the lavatory, he stayed in his bed most of the day, sleeping a great deal of the time. After about six weeks, his condition had hardly changed at all. One day, he quite anxiously raised the fact that he was not getting any better, but his anxiety was clearly about the possibility of being sent home again. On being reassured that this was not going to happen, he asked if he was dying. He was told that no one expected him to die for several months yet, but that his disease could not be cured and it would eventually catch up with him. His response was very philosophical; he thought he had had a good innings. He said he had to tell his brother because he needed to make a will. He gave a rueful smile and said, 'Well, seein' as 'ow I'm only five foot tall, the coffin won't cost 'em much'.

Thomas talked a lot more over the next couple of months, recalling all manner of tales about life on the farm, about the two hundred and forty moles he had caught and skinned to make a coat for the postmistress, and how she still would not marry him! He talked about his garden and his favourite plants. He asked about the probable mode of his death once or twice, but was easily reassured by honest information.

Thomas slept for longer and longer periods each day, often surprising the staff by waking up and demanding a three course breakfast in the middle of the morning. He was peacefully unconscious for nine days before he finally died. His death was as peaceful as the life which preceded it.

Joan

Joan was a surgeon who had been based at a missionary hospital in Nigeria for twenty-five years. It was on her fiftieth birthday that she diagnosed herself as having a brain tumour, after which she arranged a flight back to London. It proved to be an inoperable glioblastoma. Radiotherapy was given, but the prognosis was still thought to be very short.

Not having a home in England other than with her mother, who was far too handicapped herself to look after anyone else, Joan decided to make her home in the hospice for what time remained. At first she would go off to stay with friends for week-ends or go out to concerts or meals in the evenings. In fact she was taken to services at a local church by some of the parishioners until the week of her death.

Joan had faced up to the possible terminal nature of her disease the moment she developed a hemiparesis in Nigeria, and she had insisted on seeing her brain scan and other diagnostic test results right from the beginning. She was, therefore, aware that her days were very limited now. It hardly needs saying, in view of the nature of her work, that Joan was a committed Christian. Her faith was very much of the 'loving, forgiving God' type and she never seemed to falter in her belief at all. She was able to admit to tremendous feelings of panic when the truth had first dawned upon her. She had experienced all the physiological symptoms of panic, but even then she said that something inside her kept telling her that all would be well.

Some of her deepest fears were experienced when asleep, for on several occasions she dreamt that she had died and discovered that there was no God after all. These dreams haunted both her waking and sleeping hours for nearly two weeks, often causing her to wake up in the middle of the night terrified and trembling all over. Pastoral counselling was provided by the hospital chaplain, by Christian members of staff and by the friends who streamed in each day. Eventually the dreams ceased, and as the days passed by Joan became positively radiant with peace and joy. At one point she became rather impatient, wondering why God was keeping her hanging about for so long, but she decided there must be a purpose, that He must have more work for her to do, so she began recording her memoirs.

Joan's relationships with the other patients were a source of great pleasure and support to them all. There was nothing pious or 'holier than thou' about her; she was full of fun and vitality. She would entertain them with incredible tales of her adventures as a mission doctor. She inspired great trust in everyone, and many of the patients shared their deepest fears and worries with her. Even though facing death herself, she was able to listen attentively to their distress and give them the support that they needed, support which was so much more valuable because they knew that she really understood what it felt like to be dying.

Joan's main fears about the mode of dying were the possibility of losing her sight or her ability to communicate. Fortunately, neither of these happened and she died in a state of peaceful acceptance and joyful anticipation of what was to come.

REFERENCES

Hinton, John, *Dying.* Pelican, 1967.
Kübler-Ross, E., *On Death and Dying.* Tavistock, 1973.

Chapter 6

Pain and its Relief

WHAT IS PAIN?

'Pain' is derived from the Latin word, 'poena', meaning punishment. It is a dual phenomenon, consisting of a physiological sensation and an emotional response to the sensation. The emotional response is partly determined by the severity of the sensation, but the sociological and psychological make-up of the sufferer also play a major part.

Children usually adopt their parents' attitude to pain during the first years of life, though this is modified by personal experience of illness and pain, as well as by personality type.

The psychological component is demonstrated clearly on the battlefield or on the football pitch, where there have been many incidents of soldiers and sportsmen continuing to fight or play, quite oblivious of severe injuries. In contrast, a patient undergoing a surgical operation, which inflicts comparatively minor physical damage, may be overwhelmed with pain because his attention is so sharply focussed upon it.

The psychological component is sometimes so great that it not only affects the emotional response, but actually seems responsible for producing the physiological sensation. Although the organic origin of pain is quite apparent, in the case of a prolapsed vertebral disc or an osteoarthritic joint, for example, the psychological origin is just as clearly demonstrated in a hysterical conversion, an asthma attack or a migraine.

The sociological or cultural component can be seen in multiracial societies, such as Malaysia, where the Chinese women give birth in a silent, stoical manner, alongside the excitable and frequently distraught Malay women. Because the attitude to pain is so different, so is the way in which it is experienced and, consequently, the resulting behaviour.

So what is pain? Intense, harmful stimulation of body tissue does not necessarily result in severe pain. Pain is precisely what the patient says it is, occurring when he says it occurs and hurting as much as he says that it hurts. If a patient's pain threshold is low, due to anxiety, fear, cultural attitudes or a chronic personality disorder, the pain is just as real and should be treated as such. A low pain threshold is no excuse for inadequate pain relief. Moral judgements are often made quite unconsciously, confusing a high pain threshold with courage. It is so easy to sympathise with the brave, uncomplaining patient, but equally easy to be critical of, and brusque with, those who appear intolerant of seemingly minor pains.

In the patient suffering from a terminal illness, the physical origins of pain may be many. Invasion or obstruction of organs, vessels and bones by tumour, pressure on nerves, muscle spasms, pathological fractures, pressure sores and constipation are some of the more common ones. The fear instilled by a fatal disease, especially when it is malignant, will invariably magnify the emotional response to pain stimuli. Similar levels of pain induced in healthy volunteers will produce negligible distress, whilst those with cancer are likely to complain of severe pain. The presence of a frontal lobe cerebral tumour will occasionally result in an autoleucotomy. The consequent disappearance of any emotional response to pain can be dramatic. The stimulus remains the same, but the patient becomes quite unperturbed by it. Most pain experienced by the terminally ill is protracted, and is associated with the progression and irreversible nature of the disease. It often grows gradually more severe, expanding to occupy the patient's whole attention, isolating him in a world of pain.

Cancer causes some of the most severe pain amongst the dying. However, contrary to popular belief, the pain suffered by those with terminal malignant disease varies enormously from patient to patient. Approximately one-third never suffer anything more than discomfort, some not even that, whilst the remaining two-thirds experience a degree of pain which ranges from moderate to overwhelming. As mentioned above, this may or may not be proportional to the physical extent of the disease.

THEORIES OF PAIN MECHANISMS

It has long been accepted that the classical physiology of pain is not the complete story. The ways in which mood or culture can affect the experience of pain, perhaps more than the severity of the stimulus itself, have already been discussed. Recently, other physiological factors have been discovered which have an important bearing on the transmission and interpretation of pain. These have given rise to the 'pattern' and the 'gate control' theories. Nevertheless, it is still useful to have a basic knowledge of the classical pain pathways, as the severance or blockage of nerves is dependent upon this information. This approach is based on what is sometimes called the 'specificity' theory.

Specificity Theory
Impulses from special sensory nerve endings in the skin or muscles travel along special sensory nerve fibres until they join the posterior nerve roots. A synapse occurs in the posterior spinal ganglion. The impulse then enters the dorsal horn of grey matter in the spinal cord. At this point, these special nerves conveying impulses of pain, along with those conveying temperature and pressure, take a different pathway from those of light touch and the sense of body position. Whilst the latter ascend in the posterior columns of white matter, the former synapse in the dorsal horn of grey matter and are relayed to the opposite side of the spinal cord, left to right and right to left, as the lateral spinothalamic tract. They then ascend in the lateral columns of white matter to the thalamus, deep in the cerebral hemispheres, then out to the sensory area of the cerebral cortex where the impulses are interpreted (Figure 6.1).

The autonomic nervous system, though largely concerned with efferent nerve pathways, does play a part in the conveyance of pain from the viscera. The afferent sympathetic and parasympathetic nerves do, however, mostly use the same ascending routes as the somatic sensory nerves. Viscera are sensitive only to tension and chemical changes, with a suprising insensitivity to burning, cutting or crushing.

Although this simple theory is not the complete picture, certain small nerves are especially, if not exclusively, involved in the transmission of painful stimuli. This is demonstrated when one of the lateral spinothalamic tracts is severed, since there will be a consequent loss of pain and temperature sensitivity below the lesion on the opposite side.

Pattern Theory
This theory claims that no nerves exist specifically for the relay of pain impulses, but that the brain recognises certain patterns of information as pain. This explains how different types of sensory information interact, since they are all travelling along the same nerve fibres, and why an identical impulse may cause pain on one occasion, but not on another.

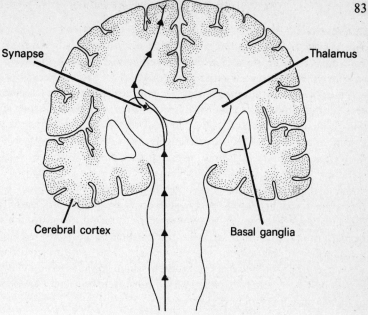

a) Cross section of cerebral hemispheres.

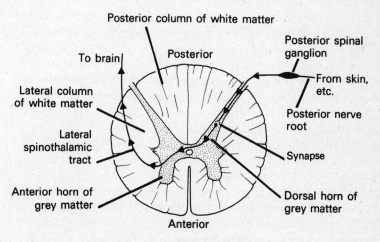

b) Cross section of spinal cord.

Figure 6.1. *Cross Sections of Cerebral Hemisphere and Spinal Cord Showing the Pathway of a Nerve Conveying Pain i.e. Specificity Theory.*

Gate Control Theory

This is based on the understanding that not all sensation from within and outside of the body is allowed to enter the brain. If this were the case, organised activity would be impossible. The 'gate' or site of control is thought to be within the substantia gelatinosa. This is the translucent grey matter which caps the dorsal horn of the spinal cord. Surprisingly, it is the stronger impulses, carried in thick nerve fibres, which appear to stimulate the cells in the substantia gelatinosa and close the gateway to the brain. Activity in small nerve fibres passes through without difficulty, however, which may explain the distress which many low-key, niggling discomforts can cause. Prolonged input by the small nerve fibres positively helps to keep the gate open, by suppressing activity in the substantia gelatinosa. In consequence these minor pains are self-perpetuating. It is thought that the gate can also be closed by descending messages from the central nervous system. This would explain why, when carrying a boiling hot soup tureen, which happens to be a valuable family heirloom, the full impact of the burning pain is not experienced until the tureen is safely deposited.

It is probable that all three theories contain a large element of truth. As yet, a complete and proven understanding of the mechanism of pain is not available. A more recent advance in research is the discovery of body opiates or, to be precise, peptides with opioid properties, known as enkephalins and endorphins. How and when these substances are released is not yet known, but it may be a clue to the efficacy of acupuncture. Opiate-receptor sites are found in those areas of the brain known to be involved with emotional behaviour, the primitive part of the thalamus, the hypothalamus, the prefrontal lobe and the limbic lobe. This would explain the profound euphoric effect of morphine. They are also found in the gut, which would explain the severity of the constipation problem in patients taking regular doses of opiates.

Another area into which research is being carried out is the apparent analgesic effect of dopamine and serotonin, two of the three substances necessary for the transmission of nerve impulses across a synapse (the other being noradrenaline). Certain drugs, such as bromocriptine (Parlodel), have been found to enhance the analgesic effect of dopamine.

These are just two examples of how an increased understanding of the mechanisms of pain can lead to future advances in pain relief.

ASSESSMENT OF PAIN

When assessing the terminally ill, they are frequently found to be so exhausted and demoralised by weeks of unrelieved pain that they are incapable of giving a clear account of its sites and severity. Consequently, it is often best if the doctor ascertains the drug and the dosage which had been previously prescribed, but proved ineffective, and gives an increased dose of the same, returning to assess the pain several hours later. If the drug is totally inadequate, however, a more suitable drug may have to be given immediately. Patients overwhelmed in this way will feel pain 'all over'. This is partly due to muscle spasm caused by the constant pain and tension.

Once the patient is more comfortable and relaxed, a detailed assessment can be made. A diagram of a body outline can be extremely useful, the patient being asked to help mark the sites of his pain on the chart (Figure 6.2). Pains shooting from one site into a limb, or over the back of the head, for example, can be indicated by arrows. If three coloured pens are supplied, the mild, moderate or severe nature of the pain at each site can be indicated. Other questions which need to be asked are, 'How long have you had your pain?', 'Does your pain limit your activity in any way?', 'Does your pain keep you awake at night?', 'How constant or variable is your pain?', 'Which movements make the pain worse?', 'Have you found anything which eases the pain?' and 'What does the pain feel like?' Preprinted charts, giving a full range of possible answers to each question, may make it easier for patients to respond accurately, particularly when trying to describe the nature of pain.

Examples of the kind of questions, and typical answers, that could be used are: *Question*—'Please tick those words which best describe your pain. It does not matter how many you tick.' *Answer*—'Throbbing, shooting, stabbing, prickling, sharp, gnawing, pulling, burning, tight, itchy, stinging, heavy, raw, numb, nauseating, pressing, cold, dull, nagging.' Or: *Question*—'Does the pain limit your activity in any way?' *Answer*—'Not at all, confined to the house most of the time, confined to the house all of the time, minimal limitation within the home, considerable limitation within the home, mainly in a chair or bed, completely bedfast.'

Once a clear picture of the pain has been gained, the pre-assessment medication should be reviewed. It is important to discover not only *how effective* the medication was, but also *how long* the relief lasted.

If a patient has a diagnosis of renal failure, motor neurone disease or

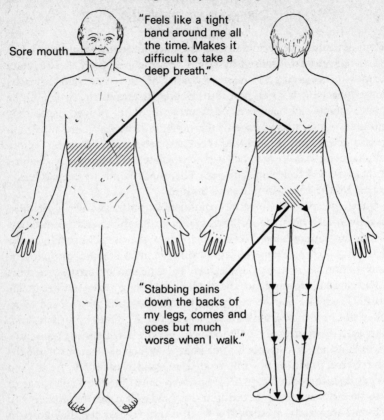

Sore mouth

"Feels like a tight band around me all the time. Makes it difficult to take a deep breath."

"Stabbing pains down the backs of my legs, comes and goes but much worse when I walk."

Figure 6.2. *The Use of a Body Chart in the Assessment of Pain.*

cancer, it does not automatically follow that these are the causes of every pain that he experiences. Dying patients are just as susceptible as anyone else, in fact more so, to pain from dental caries, peptic ulceration, haemorrhoids or constipation. Accurate diagnosis and appropriate treatment is essential. Indigestion in a patient with motor neurone disease will respond to an antacid just as well as in an otherwise healthy person. Even those pains which are caused by the main disease require careful diagnosis. Backache caused by a collapsed lumbar vertebrae in a patient with spinal metastases will need very different treatment from the backache of a patient with pancreatic carcinoma.

In addition to the patient's account of his pain, there are three other major components of the assessment. These are firstly, a detailed summary of the recent and past medical history, secondly, a thorough physical examination and thirdly, nursing observation. The latter will include observation of restlessness, range of movements and degree of mobility, mood, appetite and sleep. Many of these would have been included in the patient's own assessment, but it is always valuable to compare the patient's answers with a more objective view. Time and again, patients will understate the degree of their pain for fear of being a nuisance or appearing to lack courage. A few will overstate their case, as a result of anxiety and previous failure to obtain relief.

PAIN RELIEF

Having already appreciated that pain is a dual phenomenon, consisting of both a physiological sensation and an emotional response to the sensation, it would seem foolish to think of treating the physiological sensation alone, without any serious regard to the emotional condition of the sufferer.

Anger, depression, fear, anxiety and anticipatory grief, all common amongst the terminally ill, will intensify pain. Such emotions will magnify the way that the pain stimulus is experienced, and consequently the response to it. The first line of attack, therefore, must be to help unleash these emotions and to provide support for those who are experiencing and venting them.

Fear and anxiety are often the most difficult to overcome, since any pain experienced by a dying person will invariably produce both of these emotions. The fear and anxiety will in their turn increase the experience of, and response to, the pain stimulus. When attempting to reduce fear and anxiety, patients should be nursed in an atmosphere of calm, by staff who are caring and competent. They should be given the information which they need about their disease and the emotional support to deal with it. They will also need to feel totally accepted by those who are caring for them, and they will require the highest possible standard of physical nursing care. In this kind of environment, fear and anxiety can usually be expressed in words, tears and silent companionship, instead of pain.

Social factors may be a cause of anxiety, particularly for those with dependants. Worries about finance, about how the illness is affecting the children and if they are being properly fed, or whether an aged parent is remembering to light the gas once he has turned it on, are typical of the concerns which go round and round in a sick person's mind, aggravating every ache and pain. The organisation of practical help for the dependants may produce a marked reduction in the patient's pain.

So even before embarking upon a detailed analysis of the causes of pain, and the possible prescription of drugs, nerve blocks or surgery, for example, every dying patient must be related to as a 'whole person', each with a unique set of emotional needs.

NON-DRUG TREATMENTS OF PAIN

When confronted with a patient in pain, the instinctive and correct response is to try to relieve the pain as quickly and effectively as possible. For most doctors this will mean the prescription of drugs, as they frequently assume this to be the only channel open to them. Unfortunately, both analgesics and psychotropic drugs, the two groups most effective in pain relief, have serious side-effects; these include some loss of mental acuity, or clouding of consciousness, however minimal. This may produce an initial euphoria, but more often will heighten feelings of loss of control and may contribute to an overall sense of demoralisation and depression.

Nevertheless, drugs do play a vital role in the control of pain in terminal illness. A great deal of the more severe pain seems amenable to no other form of treatment. The automatic use of drugs as the first and only line of attack should be discouraged, however, in view of the wide variety of non-drug treatments which are available.

The following section outlines the conventional non-drug treatments, such as surgery and radiotherapy, as well as a few of the less commonly accepted ones. The wider use of some of the latter, such as acupuncture, hypnotherapy and psychoprophylaxis, are dependent upon the learning of new skills by both doctors and nurses.

Many of the non-drug treatments for pain are not alternatives to drugs, but extremely valuable adjuncts. They will not only enhance the use of conventional drugs, but may also reduce their required dosage. As with drug-therapy, not all non-drug treatments will be suitable for all dying patients with pain, and several treatments may have to be tried before the most beneficial one is found.

Diversional Therapy
Even when patients are seriously ill, it is often useful to provide some diversional therapy. The idea behind this is not to prevent them from ever thinking about their situation, but to ensure that they are not left

without any other alternative, twenty-four hours of the day, and to relieve boredom.

Patients who are very weak, or whose cerebration and coordination are affected by their disease or medication, will require great sensitivity from the occupational therapist. They will need to be given tasks which are considerably more simple than their previous level of capability. Because this can be both painful and worrying, a skilful therapist will encourage the patient to attempt crafts which he has never tried before. In this way the comparison with previous standards is not so obvious. Even the simplest item, such as a knitted dish-cloth, can give great satisfaction as long as it is something which will be useful. To expect someone to spend their time making something which is neither attractive nor useful is clearly insulting.

Diversional therapy does not only consist of crafts. A good supply of games, books and magazines, a radio and television, visitors and ward activities all divert the patient's attention from his pain. As a result, the actual sensation of pain may be lessened.

As always, the best way of finding out how to meet a patient's needs is to ask him. His special interest may be filling in betting forms and following the races, wood carving, putting the family snaps into albums or sketching the ward. Since the great majority of the occupational therapist's time will be spent with those capable of some degree of rehabilitation, the nursing staff should be prepared to play a role in discovering such interests and doing all they can to accommodate them.

Simple Physical Means of Relieving Pain
Some pains can be alleviated by the most simple medical or nursing techniques. Positioning a patient in such a way that pressure is relieved from sensitive areas is probably the most useful. Metastatic deposits in the spine, particularly when there is any vertebral collapse, must be one of the most common and severe causes of positional pain in cancer patients. In such cases, every effort should be made to keep the spine immobile. If the lesions are in the cervical or thoracic spine, an adjustable hinged bed, which allows the patient to be sat up whilst keeping the head, neck and back supported at all times, will be a great help in relieving both pain and the fear of pain. The base of these beds consists of two sections hinged together, allowing both the foot and the head to be elevated by turning a handle or using a foot-pump (Figure 6.3). When even this amount of movement produces paid, a Stryker frame or body splint may be necessary. The lighter materials now available are more comfortable than the old-fashioned plaster of Paris

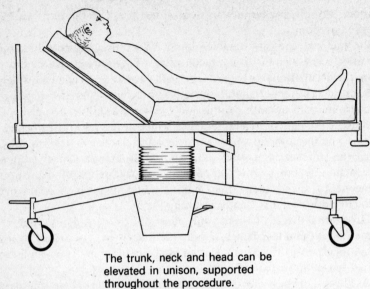

The trunk, neck and head can be
elevated in unison, supported
throughout the procedure.

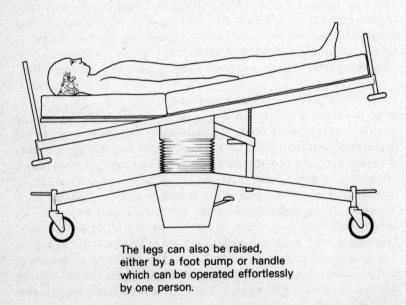

The legs can also be raised,
either by a foot pump or handle
which can be operated effortlessly
by one person.

Figure 6.3. *The Use of an Adjustable, Hinged Bed.*

jackets. If the splint is split down either side, the upper half can be removed after turning. Swollen limbs are always more comfortable when elevated, and morning headaches caused by raised intracranial pressure can be eased considerably by raising the head of the bed at night. (For the more general principles of positioning, see page 165.)

Local application of heat seems to soothe both body and mind. A hot water bottle or heat pad, a 'deep heat' spray or an infra-red lamp applied to a tender area where the muscles are in spasm, will sometimes prove as effective as an analgesic. Ice packs applied to hot, inflamed areas causing pain will be similarly effective.

Splints or skin traction may be usefully employed to immobilise a fractured limb, or one in which nerves are compressed on movement. Some fractures, however, will necessitate surgical pinning.

Aspiration of fluid from the pleural and peritoneal cavities can greatly relieve the discomfort of gross distension, as well as dyspnoea and other symptoms.

It may be necessary to encourage patients to change their habits a little, in order to ease some kinds of pain. This may mean sitting rather than standing when shaving or doing the ironing; it may mean getting a gas fire installed to avoid carrying heavy buckets of coal, or it may mean converting the living room into a bedroom to avoid climbing stairs. Sometimes, more serious changes in life-style are called for, such as giving up a physically arduous job.

Radiotherapy

Even when a patient is terminally ill, radiotherapy may be useful in pain relief, particularly for the irradiation of bony metastases. This may be possible in a single shot, but if a higher dose is required, the treatment may be spread over a period of two weeks in order to keep side-effects to a minimum. These can include severe fatigue and weakness, anorexia, nausea and vomiting, diarrhoea, burns, alopecia and mouth ulcers, as well as depression of the bone marrow. However, these symptoms rarely occur with any severity following a short course of treatment aimed at relieving pain only.

Surgery

Two of the ways in which surgery is occasionally employed for the relief of pain are the removal of endocrine glands and the severance of nerves.

A hypophysectomy, adrenalectomy, orchidectomy or oophorectomy may be performed on patients with hormone-dependent tumours. In many cases, this not only slows down the progress of the disease but also alleviates pain, particularly in the bones, in a way that is not fully understood. The relief is negligible in some patients and dramatic in others. These operations are increasingly being replaced by radiotherapy and cryosurgery, which can ablate the glands with far less trauma. Pituitary glands are also being injected with alcohol, and aminoglutethimide is being prescribed to curtail the production of hormones medically.

Neurosurgical procedures include cordotomy or percutaneous cordotomy (the division of the lateral spinothalamic tract), rhizotomy (the cutting of nerve roots), the destruction of the thalamus, and leucotomy. The neurosurgeon may also perform hypophysectomies. All of these neurosurgical procedures are uncommon.

The general surgeon will occasionally be asked to help in the relief of pain from abdominal obstruction, an abscess, or a fistula.

If a large metastatic deposit in a long bone is causing pain on weight-bearing, has eroded fifty per cent or more of the cortex of the bone, and is very likely to result in a pathological fracture, it may be appropriate for an orthopaedic surgeon to insert an intra-medullary pin prophylactically. This would help to relieve pain, improve mobility and avoid the trauma of a spontaneous fracture.

Cryoanalgesia
Cryoanalgesia is a technique in which extremely low temperatures are used to alleviate pain, by blocking peripheral nerves or destroying nerve endings. The equipment used consists of a cryoprobe, which has an inner tube and a fine nozzle through which gas is delivered under high pressure. When the probe is applied to living tissue, heat is extracted from it, thus producing a rapid drop in temperature. The formation of intracellular and extracellular ice causes a local destruction of the cells. Cryoanalgesia causes minimal bleeding and additional pain, and has been found to be extremely valuable in the treatment of head and neck cancer pain, particularly when facial neuralgia is a problem.

Barbotage and Ice Cold Saline
In performing barbotage, a lumbar puncture needle is inserted into the subarachnoid space and approximately 20ml of cerebrospinal fluid (CSF) are withdrawn. This is then pumped in and out, fifteen to twenty times, under pressure.

Another pain-relieving procedure is the withdrawal of 80ml of CSF and the injection of 80ml of normal saline at 0°C into the subarachnoid space. This is always performed under general anaesthesia as it is so painful. These treatments are both thought to relieve pain by damaging the lateral spinothalamic tracts. The headache experienced by many patients following these procedures is very severe and protracted. In addition, the long-term relief of pain is unreliable.

Acupuncture Analgesia
Acupuncture has received a great deal of publicity in the West in recent years and there are an increasing number of practitioners. There is an initial reduction in pain in eighty per cent of the cases treated and yet its principles are very alien to the Western understanding of anatomy, physiology and disease.

Acupuncture is based on the Chinese concept of 'Ch'i . . . energy', which is believed to flow through twelve channels, known as meridians, linking the internal organs of the body. The acupuncture points, where the needles are inserted, are the points at which the meridians lie near to the surface of the body.

Acupuncturists believe that all illness is the result of stress and its interference with the energy flow. Once this happens, they believe that the body becomes susceptible to infection and other diseases. In treating pain, the acupuncturist will select the particular points on the meridian pathway at which he believes stress caused the initial interference of the flow. Needles are then inserted, and are sometimes vibrated or twisted around.

Some believe that the ensuing pain relief is due to the stimulation of thick nerve fibres and the consequent closing of the gate in the dorsal horn of the spinal cord, whilst others think it is due to stimulation of the production of body opiates.

Counter Pains
In the previous description of the gate control theory (page 84), it was seen how impulses travelling along the fine nerves were likely to be self-perpetuating, keeping the gate open, whilst impulses travelling in the thick nerve fibres were likely to cause the closing of the gate. This partly explains why rubbing a painful area brings relief. The rubbing stimulates the thick fibres, thus closing the gate.

Transcutaneous nerve stimulation is the method of pain relief based on this theory. Low intensity electrical stimulators are now available. The electrodes are placed either on the trigger zones (those sites which when palpated induce the pain) or else on the main routes of the peripheral nerves supplying the painful region. The stimulation varies from a thumping sensation to a tingling sensation. This is regulated to attain the maximum degree of comfort and pain relief.

Many patients with paraplegia experience pain at the margin between their normal and numbed skin. Transcutaneous nerve stimulators are sometimes particularly effective in relieving this.

Psychoprophylaxis

Although psychoprophylaxis is more frequently associated with the pains of childbirth, it is equally applicable to any other form of pain. Techniques of breathing at differing depths and speeds, the relaxation of muscles to maintain a good supply of blood to the painful area, and the ability to keep the attention on things other than pain, can be used by the terminally ill with great benefit. The teaching of these basic principles should be included in the nursing care of all patients with chronic pain.

Hypnosis

The attitude of someone suffering from protracted pain is usually one of anxiety, fear, depression and helplessness. This attitude of mind undoubtedly exacerbates the pain, but to change it to one of confidence and control in a patient who is fully alert is virtually impossible. However, encouragement towards a more positive attitude given to someone in a hypnotic state can be extremely successful.

The hypnotic state is characterised by decreased peripheral awareness and increased focal awareness. The patient is not asleep, but in an altered state of awareness in which he has a heightened level of suggestibility. The hypnotherapist does not claim to have any supernatural powers, but rather the knowledge of an easily-learned technique. Before hypnotising the patient, he will get to know him extremely well, taking a detailed social and medical history and giving a clear account of the nature of hypnosis. His conversation will then gradually take on a slow, repetitive form and his voice will become more gentle. Dreamlike pictures will be painted in words, and an object may be swung rhythmically within the patient's gaze.

All suggestions made by the therapist must be open-ended, and rigid instructions avoided. As a result, the pain may decrease or even go away completely. It is important for patients to retain some awareness of their pain, because of its protective function as a warning system.

An increasing number of doctors, nurses and psychiatrists are learning the skills of hypnosis, and some are teaching self-hypnosis as an adjunct to other methods of pain relief.

Yoga

Those who practise yoga are able to achieve an extremely high level of muscular relaxation. All pain produces muscle spasm, both locally around the focus of the pain and generally, if unrelieved for any length of time, as an overall increase in muscle tension. Any practice which systematically relaxes every muscle of the body is therefore a most useful tool. Fortunately, yoga classes are now widely available.

Before attending a yoga class, all patients should consult their doctor as to its advisability. Occasionally, where nerve compression or disease of the bones or joints, especially the spine, are present, certain yoga positions will need to be avoided.

Meditation

Although meditation is traditionally viewed in connection with religious contemplation, it can also be used in a quite secular manner, as a technique for achieving profound physical and psychological relaxation. It is possible to use this technique to achieve a state of consciousness in which the mind is fully alert and yet the activity within the brain is less than when in a deep sleep. By meditating regularly, usually twenty minutes twice daily, it has been shown that stress can be neutralised. There is a great deal of physiological evidence of this process. The metabolic rate, pulse rate, respiratory rate and blood pressure drop dramatically, skin and muscle tension is reduced, sweating is diminished and the level of lactic acid is lowered considerably. Electroencephalogram tracings show a synchronisation and regularity of cerebral activity quite unlike those seen in sleep or any other state.

Transcendental meditation is one of the most popular, non-religious forms of meditation, and is increasingly recommended by doctors for those suffering from the more obviously stress-related diseases, such as asthma or hypertension. Few things give rise to greater stress than fatal illness and pain. The pain threshold can become a great deal higher by neutralising stress with this technique, greatly reducing the need for tranquillising and pain-killing drugs.

Biofeedback

Biofeedback is a means of increasing conscious awareness of the internal functioning of the body. By becoming sufficiently in touch, certain activities of the autonomic nervous system can be controlled by the conscious mind. These can include the blood pressure, heart rate, respiratory rate and both skin and muscle tension. These are some of the functions affected by the 'fight or flight' response and those which are stimulated by pain. If this response can be consciously inhibited, the pain will be lessened considerably. When first acquiring biofeedback skills, electrical recording devices are used to measure changes in the various autonomic activities.

Biofeedback is still in the early stages of development, but it is being taught in several hypertension and pain clinics.

THE USE OF DRUGS

The great majority of patients who are dying and in pain are treated with drugs alone, even though it will by now be apparent that this should not be the case. But drugs are certainly the most effective single weapon against pain that we have at present, so it is vital that they are used with maximum skill.

WHERE DRUGS WORK

The site at which pain-relieving drugs work varies widely. Local anaesthetics, anti-inflammatory agents and mild analgesics, such as paracetamol and aspirin, act on the peripheral, sensory nerve endings. Local anaesthetics are also used in blocking the nerves relaying pain at almost any point along a nerve root, or in the spinal cord itself. Narcotic drugs, even the mildest, such as codeine, and psychotropic drugs have their effect on the cerebral cortex, affecting mood and the emotional response to the pain stimuli. Narcotic analgesics also have an effect on the thalamus (Figure 6.4).

ESSENTIAL PRINCIPLES IN THE USE OF ANALGESICS

When using analgesic drugs in terminal care, there are four essential principles. Firstly, since almost all pain will be of a chronic nature, medication must be given prophylactically, at regular, frequent intervals. Secondly, the pain-fear cycle must be broken; an adequate dose of a sufficiently potent drug must be found to eliminate· pain completely, or at least to the patient's satisfaction, with the minimum degree of drowsiness. Thirdly, a detailed and accurate diagnosis of the causes of the pain must be made, so that the most appropriate analgesic can be selected. Fourthly, the pain and medication will need to be reviewed frequently, because new pains may develop, existing pains may worsen, or the reduction of fear and anxiety may lessen the pain considerably.

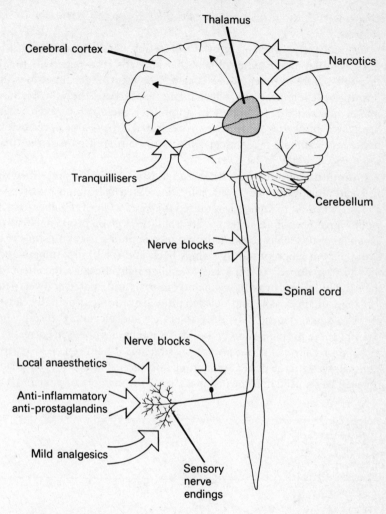

Figure 6.4. *The Sites in the Nervous System where Pain-Relieving Drugs Act.*

The use of strong, narcotic drugs is usually essential when dying patients are in severe pain, and yet there is a reluctance on the part of some doctors to prescribe them, as well as of some nurses to administer them. Fears of hastening death, fears of causing addiction and the need for escalating doses, deficient or inaccurate knowledge about the use of narcotics, and the amount of time and trouble involved in recording and checking the administration of controlled drugs, are just a few of the reasons.

Consequently, when doctors do prescribe narcotic analgesics, the dose is often inadequate. When this happens, the pain will break through before the next dose is due. The returning pain causes an upsurge of fear and anxiety, which further exacerbates the pain. Because nurses are similarly reluctant to administer these drugs, even when adequate analgesics have been prescribed, they are nevertheless frequently withheld if a patient appears to be free of pain at the time when they are due to be given.

In both the above cases, when an inadequate dose is prescribed or when administration is delayed, pain is increased by fear and anxiety. As a result, the dose of analgesic required for relief will be far higher than it would have been if an adequate dose had been given prophylactically. This higher dose may result in drowsiness, euphoria, or confusion. The dying patient who constantly swings back and forth, first in pain and then feeling 'doped', is still a sadly familiar sight. Because the effect of the drug in taking away the pain and misery is anticipated and yearned for, inadequate dosage and delayed administration can actually cause phsychological dependency, drug tolerance and escalating doses.

All of these problems can be avoided if analgesics are used correctly. Although total relief is not always possible, most pain can be lessened significantly with the patient remaining fully alert. The dose of analgesic can even be reduced in some instances, once the memory of pain and its

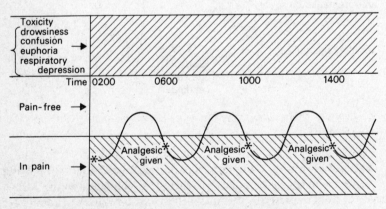

a) The prescription of inadequate doses of analgesic.

Figure 6.5. *The Different Consequences of Analgesics Used Incorrectly and Correctly.*

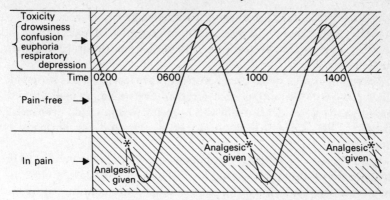

b) The delayed administration of analgesic.

associated fear begin to subside and confidence in the effectiveness of the drugs is established (Figure 6.5).

The severity of the pain and the quality of life should be the only factors which are considered when prescribing drugs for the terminally ill. Unfounded fears about hastening death or causing addiction should never be allowed to hinder adequate pain control. Although physical dependency will occur, psychological dependency is rare when narcotics are used correctly in the treatment of severe pain. Even withdrawal of

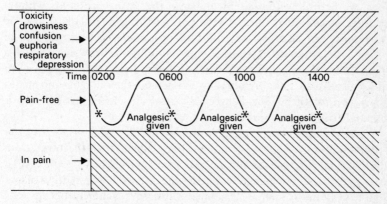

c) The prophylactic administration of analgesic in adequate dosage.

the drugs need not be a problem in the great majority of cases. If a nerve block, for instance, effects a dramatic cessation of pain, it will be possible to reduce, or even gradually to discontinue the drug altogether, without any harm.

Even the highest doses of narcotic drugs are less likely to shorten life than the emotional and physical stress of overwhelming pain. Indeed, there is strong evidence from the hospices to show that pain relief prolongs life, since the ability to sleep, rest and eat normally is recovered.

On admission to hospital, any patient whose drug regime is felt to be inadequate or unsuitable should be treated with great care. Unless the pain is entirely out of control, it is usually best to continue using the familiar drugs for at least twenty-four hours. The upheaval and loss of security caused by the admission will soon pass, and the patient's confidence and trust may be won. Meanwhile, familiar drugs, in which the patient may have some faith, should not be withheld. If necessary, more appropriate drugs can be added, in small doses, to the existing regime. Once the pain is relieved and trust has been earned, there will be no problem at all in discontinuing the ineffective medication. Of course, many patients have suffered so much pain for so long that, by the time they reach hospital, they are longing for someone to try something new. If handled sensitively, the admission itself will in many cases reduce the level of anxiety so rapidly that the pain, too, will be diminished.

When pain is not very severe, it is often better to achieve pain control gradually, beginning with relief at rest and a good night's sleep. This will improve morale and thereby increase the pain threshold, without causing severe drowsiness. Relief of pain during the day and on movement can be attempted a little later., Some patients may opt to retain a little pain on movement, thus avoiding the drowsiness which a higher dose of analgesic might cause. It is important that they are given this choice and are not pressured to accept what their doctors and nurses think best for them. This is especially relevant when a patient's work demands deep concentration.

When treating severe pain, however, the aim will be to find the optimum dose of analgesic, as quickly as possible. This is the lowest dose at which pain is relieved for at least four hours. Most people dislike taking any form of medication, and a time interval between doses of less than four hours is seen as an unacceptable encroachment on life.

A great deal of pain can be borne if the limit of its duration is known in advance. But constant, severe pain, and pain which occurs so frequently or regularly that it can be anticipated, are soon compounded by fear, anxiety and depression. This combination is overwhelming and can completely demoralise the sufferer. When treating a patient with overwhelming pain, relief must be obtained as soon as possible. This may necessitate hourly or two-hourly injections for a short period, until it is overcome, and the addition of an anxiolytic drug will almost always be required. Fear of over-sedating the patient is neither unusual nor suprising, since most people have seen patients over-sedated in normal hospital practice. In this instance, however, it is usually unfounded. After a long period of overwhelming pain, the patient will certainly be suffering from extreme exhaustion, and several hours' sleep can do nothing but good. Once the pain has been under control for a day or two, it will almost certainly be possible to reduce the dose considerably, and very often to convert to oral administration, as in the management of severe pain.

When a patient has lost consciousness in the terminal phase, or earlier in cases of cerebral tumours, it is not reasonable to assume that his awareness of pain has diminished, simply because he no longer has any means of communicating it. The same dose of analgesic should be continued regularly until the patient dies. The reasoning behind this should be explained to relatives, who are frequently suspicious of the injections, possibly fearing that euthanasia is being practised.

The pains of terminal disease can be considered under the headings of mild, moderate, severe and overwhelming, whilst others will be described as specific, because their treatment is rather different to that of most other pain. The classification of pain into different degrees of severity is dictated neither by its cause nor by the patient's response, but simply by the potency of the analgesic required to relieve it. Pain which can be alleviated by aspirin is thereby classified as mild pain. Pain which can only be relieved by narcotic analgesic is severe pain. The least potent drugs should always be tried first, and only if these prove ineffective should stronger ones be used.

RELIEF OF MILD PAIN

The following are some of the drugs of choice in the treatment of mild pain.

Acetylsalicylic acid tabs. ii-iii (600-900mg) 4 hourly
Aspirin may be taken in the traditional tablet form, as enteric-coated tablets, microencapsulated, in soluble form or combined with an

antacid. As the higher dose is often necessary, preparations which lessen the likelihood of dyspepsia or ulceration are valuable.

Paracetamol tabs. ii (1g) 4 hourly
For patients who find chalky tablets difficult to swallow, paracetamol is available in soluble form.

Benorylate (Benoral) tabs. ii (1.5g) t.d.s. or 5ml of the suspension (2g) b.d.
Benorylate is an ester of aspirin and paracetamol. A 2g dose is equipotent to approximately 1g of aspirin plus 1g of paracetamol. Its prolonged action and low incidence of gastric irritation make Benoral a useful preparation, but its high cost may be prohibitive.

RELIEF OF MODERATE PAIN

Morphine or diamorphine, taken orally, are usually the most effective drugs in the treatment of moderate pain. Because of their importance in terminal care, their use is described in a separate section (see page 106).

The following are some of the other drugs which are suitable for the treatment of moderate pain.

Dextropropoxyphene (Depronal S.A.) caps. i-ii (150-300 mg) 4-8 hourly

Dextropropoxyphene napsylate 50mg + aspirin 500mg (Napsalgesic) tabs. i-ii 4-8 hourly

Dextropropoxyphene hydrochloride 32.5 mg + paracetamol 325mg (Distalgesic) tabs. ii 4 hourly

Codeine phosphate tabs. i-ii (30-60mg) 4 hourly
This is particularly effective in the relief of headaches caused by raised intracranial pressure, but like all codeine compounds it causes severe constipation, and additional aperients may be necessary.

Codeine phosphate 8mg + aspirin 500mg (Codis) tabs. i-ii 4 hourly
Codeine is more potent than the antipyretics, having similar properties to morphine, though less than one-eighth of its analgesic properties. Combined with aspirin, it provides relief that cannot be obtained with tolerable doses of either drug alone, due to their side-effects of peptic ulceration and constipation.

Dihydrocodeine tartrate (D.F. 118) tabs. i-ii 30-60mg 4 hourly
This is another effective analgesic, but is renowned for its constipating property.

It should be noted that pentazocine hydrochloride has been found to be unsuitable for the treatment of protracted pain. When taken orally, 50mg is less potent than two tablets of codeine plus aspirin. Higher doses given regularly over a period of several weeks produce an unacceptable level of side-effects, such as nausea, vomiting, diarrhoea, dizziness, nightmares, hallucinations and dysphoria. Pentazocine is non-addictive and is, therefore, useful for short-lived pain which is not very severe, particularly post-operative pain.

RELIEF OF SEVERE PAIN

The drugs of choice in severe, protracted, cancer pain are morphine or diamorphine. Because of their importance in terminal care, their use is described in a separate section (see page 106). There are several other narcotic drugs, however, which fill a very definite role in the control of severe pain. These are listed in order of analgesic potency in Table 6.1.

Dipipanone and Cyclizine (Diconal) tabs. i-ii 4 hourly
Each tablet contains dipipanone 10mg and cyclizine 30mg. This is a useful combination for home management, with a fairly potent analgesic and an effective anti-emetic, both incorporated in one small tablet. If a dose higher than 20mg of dipipanone is required four hourly, the treatment should be changed as more than 60mg of cyclizine may cause unnecessary drowsiness or, occasionally, severe agitation and fits.

Papaveretum (Omnopon) tabs. i-ii (10-20mg) 4 hourly
This is another fairly potent analgesic, available in extremely small tablets, which are especially useful for those with difficulty in swallowing.

Levorphanol (Dromoran) tabs. i-ii (1.5-3mg) 4 hourly
Like all of the narcotic analgesics available in tablet form, Dromoran is particularly useful for patients who are at home. Measuring out solutions is inconvenient for patients who are still working and it carries a far greater risk of incorrect dosage, particularly in the elderly.

Nepenthe 10% or 20% in chloroform water, 10ml 4 hourly
This is a solution of morphine and unrefined opium, often prescribed with aspirin. The ten per cent solution is particularly convenient to use as, in that dilution, it is not a Controlled Drug under the Misuse of Drugs Act.

Oxycodone pectinate (Proladone) suppositories i-ii (30-60mg) 8 hourly
These may be valuable in delaying the use of injections when vomiting prevents the oral administration of analgesics. Their prolonged action is particularly advantageous for patients at home. When converting from morphine to Proladone or vice versa, the calculation of the correct dose is straightforward, as a dose of oral morphine provides the same level of analgesia as the identical dose given rectally.

Phenazocine (Narphen) tabs. i-ii (5-15mg) 4-8 hourly
This is the most satisfactory, potent alternative to morphine, and may be administered sublingually.

Dextromoramide (Palfium) tabs. i-ii (5-10mg) 4 hourly p.r.n.
Dextromoramide has a role in the control of intermittent and short-lived pain, particularly any form of neuralgia. It may be prescribed in addition to a longer-acting analgesic and is one of the few pain-relieving drugs which are appropriately prescribed p.r.n. in terminal care.

The drug is correspondingly unsuitable for the protracted pain from which many dying patients suffer. So often, patients taking it are admitted to hospital with their doctor's letter describing them as being 'addicted', 'clock watchers', 'difficult' or to be 'taking them like smarties'. The reason why these phrases are so common is that the drug is very quick-acting and reaches a high pinnacle of pain relief rapidly, but with an effect that lasts little over two hours.

Pethidine
Pethidine has no apparent role in relieving pain in the terminally ill. Sadly, one still sees many patients who are being nursed at home receiving inadequate oral analgesia. In an attempt to 'top this up' they are frequently given an injection of pethidine, 50 or 100mg i.m., twice daily by the district nurse. As the pain relief which this provides lasts only two or three hours, the pain during the remaining eighteen hours is likely to be worsened.

Table 6.1 Oral Analgesic Equivalence (Approximations Only)

Analgesic	Dose per Tablet (or as stated)	Equipotent Dose of Morphine	Equipotent Dose of Diamorphine
Panadol (paracetamol)	500 mg	2 mg	1 mg
Distalgesic (dextropropoxyphene+ paracetamol)	32.5 mg 325 mg	3 mg	2 mg
D.F. 118 (dihydrocodeine)	30 mg	5 mg	3 mg
Diconal (dipipanone) (30 mg cyclizine)	10 mg	5 mg	3 mg
Omnopon (papaveretum)	10 mg	5 mg	3 mg
[1]Fortral (pentazocine)	50 mg	8 mg	5 mg
[2]pethidine	50 mg	6 mg	4 mg
[3]Physeptone (methadone)	5 mg	15 mg	10 mg
Dromoran (levorphanol)	1.5 mg	8 mg	5 mg
Nepenthe 10% (morphine + opium)	10 ml	12 mg	8 mg
[4]Palfium (dextromoramide)	5 mg	15 mg	10 mg
Proladone (oxycodone pectinate)	One suppository 30 mg	20 mg	13 mg
Narphen (phenazocine)	5 mg	25 mg	16 mg

1) Pentazocine is not a potent analgesic and high doses produce severe side-effects.
2) Pethidine is too short-acting to be useful in terminal care.
3) Methadone has a prolonged plasma half-life leading to accumulation.
4) Dextromoramide is very potent but very short-acting.

Linctus of methadone hydrochloride (Physeptone linctus) 2mg in 5ml solution, 5-20ml 4-8 hourly
This is a useful preparation combining the properties of a cough suppressant and an analgesic in a linctus. It is often prescribed effectively for patients with tumours of the lung.

RELIEF OF OVERWHELMING PAIN

Morphine and diamorphine are the drugs of choice in the treatment of overwhelming pain. Because of their importance in terminal care, their use is described in a separate section (following). The only other useful drug is methadone.

Methadone hydrochloride (Physeptone) 5-200mg 4-8 hourly
The plasma half-life of methadone is more than seventy hours and, for this reason, it does have an occasional use in young patients with overwhelming pain. It is not suitable for the treatment of older patients, because of the danger of respiratory depression. In most countries, including the United States of America and Canada, the medicinal use of diamorphine (heroin) is restricted far more tightly than in Britain, and methadone is therefore used as the best available alternative. Methadone is a synthetic narcotic and is less dangerously addictive than morphine or diamorphine.

MORPHINE AND DIAMORPHINE

Morphine and diamorphine are the two most valuable and effective drugs in relieving the pains of terminal illness. Crude opium is obtained from poppy seeds; if the chief, active ingredient of opium is isolated morphine is produced, named after Morpheus, the god of sleep. Diamorphine, or heroin as it is commonly known, is a synthetic narcotic very similar to morphine. Weight for weight, diamorphine is half as strong again as morphine when taken orally, i.e. 2mg diamorphine is as potent as 3mg morphine. But diamorphine is rapidly converted to morphine in the blood and their efficacies have been found to be identical when given orally, intramuscularly, subcutaneously or per rectum. It is, therefore, not particularly important which substance is used, unless it is given intravenously, in which case diamorphine has an earlier onset of action, is more sedating and causes less vomiting than morphine.

ADMINISTRATION OF MORPHINE/DIAMORPHINE

Morphine/Diamorphine in solution
Morphine and diamorphine should be administered orally, whenever possible, as many people find suppositories distasteful and injections

frightening and painful (they can also damage tissue, see page 108). The ideal preparation is a solution of diamorphine hydrochloride or morphine sulphate in chloroform water, the traditional Brompton's cocktail (containing diamorphine or morphine, cocaine, alcohol, syrup or honey and chloroform water) no longer being considered advisable for several reasons. If a higher dose of the analgesic component was needed, the dose of cocaine and alcohol was inevitably increased at the same rate, usually quite inappropriately. The routine use of cocaine is not advisable, as it may cause agitation, confusion or hallucinations, particularly in the elderly. Even in younger patients, the tranquillising effect of the morphine or diamorphine is often desirable and a stimulant may be quite unsuitable. Even alcohol is better when added by the patient himself, according to his individual taste. Alcohol will 'burn' damaged mucosa and many patients prefer a dash of fruit juice. The routine addition of a phenothiazine to the cocktail, as a tranquilliser and anti-emetic, is also ill-advised, as the individual requirements vary so widely, with many patients needing none at all.

Solutions of morphine or diamorphine in chloroform water can be given in doses ranging from 2.5mg q.d.s. for the elderly bedfast patient with generalised aches and pains, to 200mg three hourly in rare cases of overwhelming pain. The great majority of patients will be pain-controlled on doses below diamorphine 40mg or morphine 60mg four hourly.

Patients receiving less than diamorphine 20mg four hourly or morphine 30mg four hourly can usually miss out one middle-of-the-night dose in order to obtain eight hours' sleep. One and a half times the normal dose may be necessary at bedtime, however. Those on higher doses tend to wake up with pain if not woken for their middle-of-the-night medication.

When using doses exceeding diamorphine 40-60mg, there is a marked drop in the proportional efficacy of the drug, probably due to incomplete absorption. For this reason, any increase in the prescription will probably need to be at least equal to a quarter of the previous dose.

When treatment with oral morphine or diamorphine is first initiated, between eighty and ninety per cent is converted by stomach and liver enzymes to morphine glucuronides, and is subsequently inactivated. As a result, the analgesic effect will be far less than would otherwise be expected. If the regular administration of morphine/diamorphine continues, however, the amount which is inactivated is gradually lowered. Consequently, in cases of severe pain, unless the patient has previously been taking an opiate, it may be necessary to give a four-hourly dose of morphine/diamorphine which is approximately three times as large as the anticipated dose, gradually reducing it after the first twelve hours. Alternatively, the anticipated dose can be given with the concurrent administration of diamorphine by injection for approximately twelve hours. Because of this initiation factor, morphine/diamorphine solutions taken orally are not suitable for the treatment of acute episodes of pain, their usefulness being confined to the treatment of protracted pain.

Controlled Release Morphine Tablets

Controlled release morphine has recently become available in 10mg and 30mg tablets, marketed as MST-10mg and MST-30mg respectively. In this form, the level of morphine in the blood remains high enough to control mild to severe pain for eight hours. This means that a patient 'stabilised' on 10mg of morphine in oral solution, four hourly, could be transferred to three tablets of MST-10mg twelve hourly. This preparation is unsuitable for use on initiation of treatment, as adequate blood levels are reached even more slowly than when using an oral solution. Since MST-10mg and MST-30mg have proved effective, trials with tablets of a higher dose are now in progress. This will make a significant contribution to home management in the future.

Morphine Suppositories

Suppositories containing 10mg, 15mg and 30mg of morphine are also available and are useful where nausea, vomiting or dysphagia are a problem. In the terminal phase, when the patient is losing consciousness, suppositories should always be tried before resorting to injections, though tenesmus or faecal leakage may curtail their use in some patients. Morphine per rectum is equipotent to morphine by mouth.

Injectable Morphine/Diamorphine

Morphine sulphate and diamorphine hydrochloride by injection are equally effective, but diamorphine has a practical advantage in that even a dose of 120mg can be dissolved in one millilitre of sterile water, whilst morphine sulphate is usually supplied as a solution of 10mg of morphine in 1ml. The size of the morphine injection makes it unacceptable to patients requiring a higher dose, and for this reason the use of diamorphine is recommended whenever injections are necessary. It is advisable to resort to injections only when pain is out of control and when it cannot be alleviated by oral or rectal administration. Many dying patients are very emaciated, so not only will frequent injections be distressing but injection sites will also soon become fibrous, bruised and painful.

Controlled Release Morphine for Injection

Ampoules of microcrystalline morphine 70.4mg per 1.1ml(Duromorph) $\frac{1}{2}$-2 ampoules t.d.s. or q.d.s. This is a sustained release, injectable form of morphine, which may be useful for the management of patients at home in severe pain.

Converting from Morphine to Diamorphine by Mouth and Injection

When converting from oral administration to subcutaneous or intramuscular, the oral to parenteral ratio of equipotency is approximately 3:1 for morphine and 4:1 for diamorphine; e.g. 30mg of morphine by mouth is equal in analgesic potency to 10mg by injection. Whilst the equipotent ratio of orally administered morphine to diamorphine is 3:2, the ratio when administered parenterally is 2:1; e.g. 30mg of morphine by mouth is equal in analgesic potency to 20mg of diamorphine by mouth, whereas 20mg of morphine by injection is equal in analgesic potency to 10mg of diamorphine by injection. Therefore, when converting from oral morphine to parenteral diamorphine, the dose is divided by six unless an increased dose is required; e.g. 60mg of morphine by mouth is equal in analgesic potency to 10mg of diamorphine by injection (Figure 6.6).

SIDE-EFFECTS OF MORPHINE/DIAMORPHINE

The most common troublesome side-effects of morphine and diamorphine are drowsiness, constipation, nausea and vomiting. Drowsiness varies enormously from person to person. It may be welcomed by some highly anxious patients, whilst those to whom reading and writing are important may be sufficiently incapacitated by it to refuse their medication. The drowsiness is always most pronounced when first beginning treatment and after an increase in the dosage. Patients should be prepared for this initiation response and be reassured that it will improve within a few days.

All patients treated with morphine or diamorphine become constipated, unless they have a colostomy or steatorrhea. This should be treated prophylactically, as described on pages 128 and 173.

Nausea and vomiting are not as common as is sometimes assumed, particularly when small doses of oral morphine or diamorphine are given. Some patients will be more susceptible than others, however, and

Oral morphine   Parenteral morphine

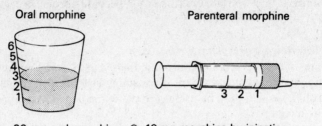

30 mg oral morphine ⌒ 10 mg morphine by injection

Oral diamorphine   Parenteral diamorphine

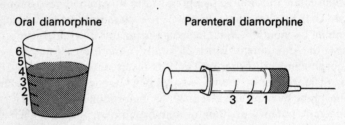

40 mg oral diamorphine ⌒ 10 mg diamorphine by injection

Oral morphine   Oral diamorphine

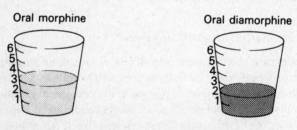

30 mg oral morphine ⌒ 20 mg oral diamorphine

Parenteral morphine   Parenteral diamorphine

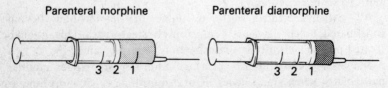

20 mg morphine by injection ⌒ 10 mg diamorphine by injection

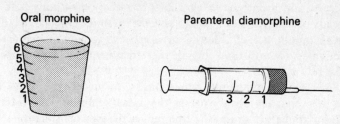

Oral morphine   Parenteral diamorphine

60 mg oral morphine ≏ 10 mg diamorphine by injection

Figure 6.6. *The Analgesic Equipotency of Morphine and Diamorphine When Given Orally or Parenterally (Approximations Only).*

most people on higher doses will need an adjuvant anti-emetic, see page 125.

Because of opiate-induced miosis, the inability to focus in order to read, write or do any kind of close work is a troublesome side-effect for some patients. Little can be done to correct this, but the use of a magnifying glass may be helpful. Some understanding opticians will go to great lengths to ameliorate the situation with spectacles, despite their knowledge that any improvement will be marginal.

Opiate-induced respiratory depression is rarely a problem in terminal care, particularly when drugs are administered orally. Anyone who is elderly or who has pulmonary oedema, and who requires a high dosage, should be observed carefully for the first twenty-four hours, however, and a supply of the antidote, naloxone (Narcan) ampoules, 0.4mg should always be available.

Intrathecal opiates have been used in an attempt to minimise these side-effects, whilst retaining the maximum benefits. Because of the presence of opiate receptors in the spine, minute doses can be given with excellent analgesic effect, but the blood level remains so low that side-effects are kept to a minimum. An indwelling, intrathecal catheter, which the patient can 'top up' himself when necessary, may be the way in which protracted, opiate-responsive pains will be treated in the future, if the danger of infection can be overcome.

RELIEF OF SPECIFIC PAIN

Bone Pain
Bone pain is one of the most common and severe pains in terminal malignancy, due to the metastatic deposits from cancer of the breast,

prostate and bronchus, in particular. Irradiation of bony lesions has already been mentioned as a valuable means of relieving pain, but when the maximum dose of radiotherapy has been given, or the patient is too debilitated to withstand any further treatment, alternative methods must be employed.

Bone pain is frequently unresponsive to opiate-type drugs alone, however high the dose, whereas the introduction of a non-steroidal, anti-inflammatory drug will often reduce the pain considerably. This is due to the resulting inhibition of the prostaglandins, a group of chemical agents present in many body tissues, which have a wide range of activity. Breast, and possibly other tumours too, secrete prostaglandins, so the level present in the body may be far higher than normal. Some prostaglandins have been found to increase the effects of pain-producing substances released from damaged or inflamed tissues, by sensitising the nerve endings. They have also been shown to induce osteolysis.

Three of the most useful anti-inflammatory agents are aspirin, 600-900mg 4 hourly, phenylbutazone (Butazolidin) 100-200mg 4 hourly, and flurbiprofen (Froben) 50-100mg q.d.s. Phenylbutazone appears to be the most effective of these, but causes blood dyscrasias, marked dyspepsia and sodium and water retention, whereas flurbiprofen combines reasonable efficacy with minimal side-effects. As all anti-inflammatory drugs have serious side-effects, such as peptic ulceration, agranulocytosis and fluid retention, it is reasonable to reduce gradually and then discontinue the treatment, if no improvement in the pain has been achieved within three days.

Patients with joint pain from immobility, especially paralysis, whose sleep is severely disturbed by pain when lying down, are sometimes helped by indomethacin (Indocid) suppositories, 100mg nocte. Occasionally, these will cause irritation of the rectal mucosa and, not uncommonly, psychological effects. One incidental value of night-time indomethacin suppositories is their ability to reduce night sweats.

Some Cancer Pains

Cytotoxic chemotherapy, hormone therapy and immunotherapy all have a very limited role in terminal care. However, the pain caused by some solid tumours, particularly those which are hormone-dependent or have presented late, and the pains of multiple myeloma, the leukaemias and lymphoproliferative disorders, may be most effectively relieved by one of these treatments.

The efficacy of cytotoxic chemotherapy is dependent on its ability to destroy rapidly dividing cells. These, of course, include malignant cells, but they also include the blood cells, hair follicles and the mucosa which lines the alimentary tract. It is the damage to these which leads to the severe side-effects of nausea, vomiting, diarrhoea, anaemia, susceptibility to infection, alopecia and mouth ulcers, for example. By reducing the size of tumours, cytotoxic drugs will relieve some types of pain, but they will also prolong life. For this reason, their use must always be considered with great care, since the severity of their side-effects will sometimes make a prolongation of life undesirable.

In order to reduce the severity of the side-effects, a combination of drugs is usually used. These will all have a slightly different mode of action, producing different side-effects. Since almost all side-effects will be unacceptable in terminal care, dosages will usually be modified and only the simplest regimes will be used. Although intravenous therapy may occasionally be appropriate, oral medication will be the norm.

Bone pain produced by the metastatic deposits of breast tumours, in both pre- and post-menopausal women, is often successfully relieved by tamoxifen (Novaldex) 10mg b.d., an anti-oestrogen agent, if this form of therapy has not already been exhausted. Similarly, the bone pain resulting from primary tumours of the prostate may be relieved by stilboestrol 5-25mg t.d.s. Tumours of the endometrium can be treated with medroxyprogesterone acetate (Provera) 100mg b.d. None of these hormonal treatments has severe side-effects, and they are therefore used far more readily than cytotoxic chemotherapy.

One of the ways in which cytotoxic drugs can be beneficial in terminal care is in connection with chest aspiration and abdominal paracentesis. Following the aspiration of fluid, thiotepa or bleomycin can be injected into the cavity. This will destroy malignant cells and may also cause adhesions to form, helping to prevent the fluid from collecting again.

Gout
Gout-like pains are not unusual following radiotherapy or chemotherapy. This is caused by a high level of blood urea which occurs following cell destruction. It is usually controlled very effectively with allopurinol (Zyloric) 100mg t.d.s.

Neuralgia
Neuralgic, stabbing pains may be caused by invasion of nerves by tumour, and are especially common in head and neck malignancies. These may be helped by carbamazepine (Tegretol) 200mg q.d.s. or sodium valproate (Epilim) 200mg q.d.s.

Nerve Compression

Nerve compression pain is best relieved by prednisolone 5-10mg t.d.s., which reduces the swelling around the tumour and consequently the degree of compression.

Causalgia

Hyperaesthetic pains, which are usually experienced as a superficial burning sensation, can be treated with amitriptyline (Tryptizol) 25-100mg b.d. or mianserin (Bolvidon) 10-30mg b.d.

Post-Herpetic Neuralgia

Post-herpetic neuralgia is not uncommon amongst the terminally ill, the incidence of herpes zoster (shingles) being higher in patients receiving chemotherapy or one of the cortico-steroids. This pain is not amenable to the usual range of analgesics or nerve blocks, but it has been found to respond to amitriptyline 25-100mg b.d. or mianserin 10-30mg b.d. A lower dose is usually given in the morning and a higher dose at night.

Many other specific pains, such as the pain from a urinary tract infection, renal colic, and dyspepsia, plus their treatment, are discussed in Chapter 7.

SUPPLEMENTARY DRUG TREATMENTS

NERVE BLOCKS

Nerve blocks, infiltrations or intra-articular injections are of great value when pain is severe and localised, particularly in cases of nerve compression or where tumour has invaded a nerve plexus.

The three types of spinal injection most commonly used are extradural, subdural and intrathecal. An extradural (or epidural) injection, as used in obstetrics, is inserted into the space in the vertebral canal around the outer layer of the meninges, the dura mater. Subdural injections are inserted between the dura mater and the arachnoid mater. Intrathecal injections are inserted between the inner covering of the spinal cord, the pia mater and the arachnoid mater. This is the subarachnoid space containing cerebrospinal fluid. The latter is used more commonly in the control of cancer pain as its effect is more powerful (Figure 6.7).

There are two factors which enable the sensory nerves conveying pain to be blocked by spinal injections, whilst leaving the motor nerves intact. The first of these is that the most troublesome pain sensations are

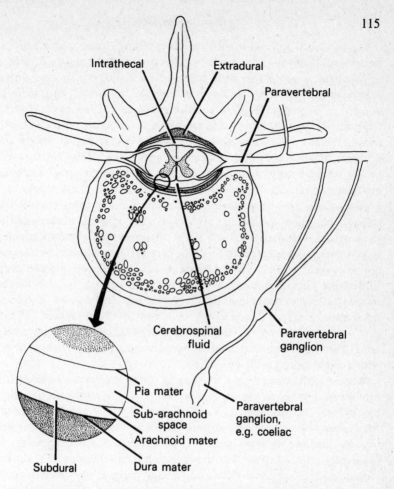

Figure 6.7. *Cross Section of a Vertebra, the Spinal Cord and a Nerve Root, Showing the Sites Where Nerve Blocks are Performed.*

carried in the smallest nerve fibres. These are damaged by neurolytic agents more severely and in greater numbers than the larger motor and sensory nerve fibres. This degree of selectivity, however, is only completely certain in extradural injections. The second factor is the position of the sensory and motor nerve roots. When intrathecal injections are performed, a solution heavier than the CSF is always used. Consequently, by lying the patient flat on his back, the neurolytic solution will concentrate around the posterior part of the spinal cord, where the sensory nerve roots emerge, leaving the motor nerve roots, which emerge from the front of the spinal cord, unaffected.

Initially, an injection with a short-acting local anaesthetic is performed in most cases. If this is effective, and the degree of motor impairment is acceptable, it is followed by a similar injection with a longer-acting solution. Accidental damage to bowel and bladder control, or even paraplegia, are not uncommon. If these are produced, temporarily, by the short-acting anaesthetic, the patient is then able to make a realistic decision about whether he is prepared to accept the possible consequences of a more permanent block. Many patients will prefer to cope with their pain, despite the inadequacy of systemic analgesics, than face the possible consequences of a nerve block.

Blocks can also be performed on sensory nerve roots outside the spinal cord. These include the thirty-one pairs of spinal nerves and the twelve pairs of cranial nerves. The spinal nerves divide into six groups, five of which join together to form the cervical, brachial, lumbar, sacral and coccygeal plexus. Nerve blocks are also performed at these sites. The twelve pairs of thoracic nerves do not form a plexus, but become the intercostal nerves supplying the intercostal muscles and ribs. These are frequently blocked successfully in cases of lung cancer. When performing plexus blocks, damage to motor nerve fibres is extremely hard to avoid, for which reason they are always preceded by an injection with a short-acting local anaesthetic.

When pain is caused by stretching of the liver capsule, a pancreatic tumour or damage to any other organ or viscera, sympathetic ganglion blocks may be performed. Visceral pain is often poorly localised, sometimes referred to a far distant site. Some of these idiosyncrasies become familiar to most nurses. The pain of a diseased appendix is frequently referred to the left inguinal fossa; gall bladder pain almost always radiates around the lower costal margin; duodenal pain is generally referred to the shoulders; pancreatic pain is usually experienced as a boring sensation in the middle of the back, and cardiac muscle pain frequently radiates down the left arm. These patterns are very variable, however, and can sometimes be misleading.

The most common sites for performing sympathetic nerve blocks are the stellate ganglion, which supplies the blood vessels of the upper limbs, the heart, bronchi and lungs, the coeliac axis ganglion, which supplies the stomach, liver, pancreas and kidney, and the lumbar sympathetic chain, which supplies the blood vessels of the lower limbs, the rectum, bladder, ureters and prostate (Figure 6.8).

Painful joints can be injected with a local anaesthetic and a steroid, with good effect. A similar combination can be used for the infiltration of peripheral nerve endings, when painful metastases have developed in soft tissues.

Local anaesthetics and other agents used in nerve blocks are:

a) Lignocaine 0.5-2%. Used for anaesthetising the skin in preparation for spinal or other nerve blocks and for diagnostic purposes.

b) Bupivacaine (Marcain Plain) 0.25% or 0.5%. A moderately long-acting local anaesthetic, used to assess the effect of most blocks before even longer-acting agents are used. (Also used for intra-articular injections.)

c) Phenol 5-7.5% in glycerine. Used for most intrathecal blocks.

d) Chlorocresol 2% in glycerine. An alternative to (c).

e) Alcohol 25-100%. Used in peripheral nerve blocks; painful to inject and causes continuous erosion of the nerves. All neurolytic agents may cause gangrene if injected into an artery.

f) Aqueous phenol 5%. Used for blocking regional sympathetic nerve supplies.

g) Methylprednisolone acetate (Depomedrone) 40-80mg. Used for intra-articular injections with bupivacaine.

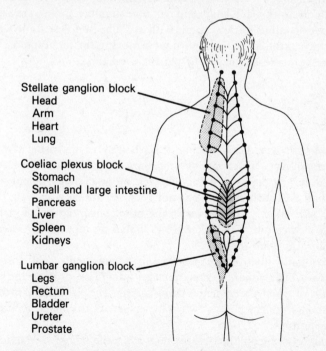

Stellate ganglion block
   Head
   Arm
   Heart
   Lung

Coeliac plexus block
   Stomach
   Small and large intestine
   Pancreas
   Liver
   Spleen
   Kidneys

Lumbar ganglion block
   Legs
   Rectum
   Bladder
   Ureter
   Prostate

Figure 6.8. *The Sites where Sympathetic Ganglion Nerve Blocks are most Commonly Performed.*

ENTONOX

Entonox is a mixture of equal parts of two gases, nitrous oxide and oxygen. Although it has long since been used in midwifery, its full potential in general medicine is only now being recognised. Entonox is effective and safe. It is very quick acting, but of short duration. Its use in cancer patients is not, therefore, in the control of chronic, continuous pains but in the control of spasmodic, severe pain.

Many patients with spinal tumours are completely free of pain when they are at rest. When they are turned for the protection of their pressure areas, however, the pain may be temporarily quite overwhelming. To give a sufficient dose of analgesic to control this intermittent pain, the patient would almost certainly be rendered extremely drowsy. If Entonox is inhaled for a short while, before and during turning, a high level of analgesia and relaxation can be achieved. It is also extremely useful when performing painful procedures, such as packing sinuses, performing certain dressings or manually emptying the bowel.

Small, portable cylinders are available. (Entonox is always stored in a blue cylinder, with a half white and half blue shoulder.) These are useful for the district nurse to carry round with her. The Bodok seal allows the patient to breathe in and out, without removing the mouthpiece. The gases are only released when the patient is inhaling.

HOMOEOPATHY

Homoeopathic remedies are being prescribed by an increasing number of doctors to treat a wide range of symptoms, including pain. The results are often very impressive. Although their mode of action is not fully understood and their efficacy has not been scientifically proven, they have no side-effects, in contrast to the now conventional, allopathic forms of medication. This factor alone should prompt further interest and exploration into their use.

Homoeopathy involves the prescription of vanishingly small doses of substances which would, if taken in larger quantities, produce the very symptoms of which the patient is complaining. The effect appears to be the stimulation of the body's own defence systems to combat the cause of the symptoms.

Although homoeopathic treatment is available within the National Health Service, it is very limited at present. It plays a far greater role in health care in France, Germany, Latin America, India and Pakistan.

THE NURSE'S ROLE

Pain can be one of the loneliest experiences, isolating the sufferer in a prison of despair. The nurse's role in administering drugs to relieve pain is an important responsibility. It is she who will observe the efficacy of the drugs and who should, therefore, be involved in decisions to increase or review them. It is the nurse who will be there when a patient becomes suddenly overwhelmed by pain. To care adequately for dying patients, especially those whose pain is severe and protracted, the nurse should be given a prescription chart which enables her to meet such an emergency immediately. She should not have to wait until a doctor can be contacted before offering some relief. Forward planning and thinking of this kind will necessarily make additional demands on the doctor's time.

An essential component in this planning is the provision of a drug chart which has one section for regular prescriptions and a second section for 'as required' drugs. Ideally, the doctor will prescribe, on the 'as required' side of the drug chart, a dose of an analgesic exceeding the regular dose in case the pain worsens, and also a parenteral alternative to the oral analgesic for emergency use in cases of extreme pain, or if the patient becomes too weak to swallow. (See Figure 6.9 overleaf.)

With this degree of autonomy, the nurse will be able to fulfil her role in meeting the challenge of pain control. Without it, impotence and frustration may lead to nurses avoiding patients in pain, or even to resenting their pleas for help.

The wider role of the nurse with regard to drugs is described on p. 123.

REFERENCES

Barnard, J. D. W. and Lloyd, J. W., 'Cryoanalgesia', in *Pain, Some Aspects*. Nursing Times Publication, 1977.

Boyd, Hamish, *Introduction to Homoeopathic Medicine*. Beaconsfield, 1981.

Eagle, Robert, *Alternative Medicine*. Futura, 1978.

Elliott, John, 'Hypnosis and Pain Relief'. *Nursing*, May 1979.

Hannington-Kiff, J. G., 'The Mechanisms of Pain'. *Nursing*, 1979.

Laurence, D. R., *Clinical Pharmacology*. Churchill-Livingstone, 1973.

Rigby, Byron, *Transcendental Meditation*. Nursing Times Reprint, 1975.

Twycross, R. G., 'Rehabilitation in Terminal Cancer Patients'. *International Rehabilitation Medicine*, June 1981.

Twycross, R. G., *Relief of Pain in the Management of Terminal Disease*, C. M. Saunders (ed.). Arnold, 1978.

Vere, D. W., 'Pharmacology of Morphine Drugs Used in Terminal Care', in *Topics in Therapeutics 4*. Pitman Medical, 1978.

Wint, Allegra, 'Acupuncture'. *Nursing*, May 1979.

PATIENT'S NAME: MARY ARNOLD (Mrs)	KNOWN DRUG SENSITIVITIES NIL												
	AS REQUIRED PRESCRIPTIONS												
DRUG (APPROVED NAME) 1. DIAMORPHINE HCl	Date	15/3	15/3										Date Cancelled
Route SC Dose 5 mg Frequency 4 hrly Start Date 9/3/83	Time	6⁰⁰	10⁰⁰										
	Dose	5mg	5mg										
SIGNATURE H.M. Grant Pharm R.B.	Given	J.P.	J.P.										
DRUG (APPROVED NAME) 2. MORPHINE SULPH.	Date	15/3											Date Cancelled 15/3/83
Route P O Dose 15-20 mg Frequency 4 hrly Start Date 9/3/83	Time	14⁰⁰											
	Dose	20 mg											
SIGNATURE H.M. Grant Pharm R.B.	Given	J.P.											
DRUG (APPROVED NAME) 3. HYOSCINE	Date												Date Cancelled
Route SC Dose 0.8 mg Frequency 4-8 hrly Start Date 9/3/83	Time												
	Dose												
SIGNATURE H.M. Grant Pharm R.B.	Given												
DRUG (APPROVED NAME) 4. MORPHINE SULPH.	Date												Date Cancelled
Route P O Dose 20-30 mg Frequency 4 hrly Start Date 15/3/83	Time												
	Dose												
SIGNATURE H.M. Grant Pharm R.B.	Given												
DRUG (APPROVED NAME) 5. DIAZEPAM	Date												Date Cancelled
Route po/IM Dose 5-10 mg Frequency 4-8 hrly Start Date 15/3/83	Time												
	Dose												
SIGNATURE H.M. Grant Pharm R.B.	Given												
DRUG (APPROVED NAME) 6.	Date												Date Cancelled
Route Dose Frequency Start Date	Time												
	Dose												
SIGNATURE Pharm	Given												
DRUG (APPROVED NAME)													Date

Figure 6.9. *The Use of a Drug Chart Demonstrating the Importance of Separate Sections: 'As Required' Drugs.*

REGULAR PRESCRIPTIONS

DRUG (APPROVED NAME)		Before food	After food	MONTH AND DATE MARCH 1983											Date Cancelled
TICK TIMES REQUIRED				9	10	11	12	13	14	15	16				

1. MORPHINE SULPH.		2														
Route po	Dose 10 mg	Frequency 4 hrly	Start Date 9/3/83	6	√		PE	PE	PE	QJ	QJ					15/3/83
				10	√		QJ	SW	MB	QJ	MB					
				14	√	QJ	QJ	SW	MB	SW	MB					
SIGNATURE H.M.Grant		Pharm. R.B.		18	√	KN	KN	QJ	KN	SW	SW					
				22	√	PE	PE	PE	QJ	QJ	PE					
2. HALOPERIDOL		2														
Route po	Dose 1.5 mg	Frequency bd	Start Date 9/3/83	6	√		PE	PE	PE	AJ	AJ	PE	SW			
				10												
				14												
SIGNATURE H.M.Grant		Pharm. R.B.		18												
				22	√		PE	PE	AJ	AJ	PE	SW	MB			
3. SOLUBLE ASPIRIN		2														
Route po	Dose 600 mg	Frequency 4 hrly	Start Date 9/3/83	6	√		PE	PE	PE	QJ	QJ	KN	KN			
				10	√		QJ	SW	MB	QJ	MB	KN	KN			
				14	√	QJ	QJ	SW	MB	SW	KN	SW	MB			
SIGNATURE H.M.Grant		Pharm. R.B.		18	√	KN	KN	QJ	KN	SW	MB	SW	KN			
				22	√	PE	PE	PE	QJ	QJ	PE	SW	MB			
4. LACTULOSE		2														
Route po	Dose 20 ml	Frequency od	Start Date 11/3/83	6												
				10												
				14												
SIGNATURE H.M.Grant		Pharm. R.B.		18												
				22	√		PE	QJ	QJ	PE	SW	MB				
5. MORPHINE SULPH.		2	√								SW				
				6	√							KN				
Route po	Dose 20 mg	Frequency 4 hrly	Start Date 15/3/83	10	√							KN				
				14	√							MB				
SIGNATURE H.M.Grant		Pharm. R.B.		18	√						SW	KN				
				22	√						SW	MB				
6.		2														
				6												
Route	Dose	Frequency	Start Date	10												
				14												
SIGNATURE		Pharm.		18												
				22												
DRUG (APPROVED NAME)		2														

Figure 6.9. *The Use of a Drug Chart Demonstrating the Importance of Separate Sections: 'Regular' Drugs.*

Chapter 7

The Medical Treatment of Other Common Symptoms

Many deaths occur suddenly and many others are preceded by a gentle weakening, with no cause for distress. Nevertheless, the multitude of symptoms which may afflict the terminally ill make gruesome reading, although the skilled use of drugs can achieve a remarkable degree of relief from almost all of them.

Some of these symptoms, when viewed alongside the awesome reality of imminent death, appear too trivial to be worth considering. Many a doctor has gaped in disbelief at the terminally ill patient who seems totally preoccupied with his constipation or oral thrush, whilst relatively unperturbed about his prognosis. This may be part of the denial process; anxiety about the future being misplaced onto something which is less frightening to contemplate. There is no doubt, however, that several minor symptoms can cause just as much distress as one major one. This can be partly explained by the gate control theory of pain transmission (page 84).

Contrary to popular belief, few terminally ill patients are still expecting their doctors to cure them. What they do need and expect is continuing involvement, a deepening relationship and conscientious attention to symptom control, however trivial the symptoms may appear to be. The doctor who is prepared and able to meet these needs will find that he is no longer overwhelmed by feelings of failure, uselessness and embarrassment. When someone dies after a terminal illness, during which his symptoms have been well-managed and both patient and relatives have received the emotional support which they needed, their doctor has every right to feel satisfied with his achievement.

When relieving symptoms, it is as essential as in any other area of medicine to diagnose the underlying cause before initiating treatment. The only difference in terminal care is that diagnoses should be made from clinical examination and scrutiny of the medical history, avoiding investigations whenever possible. If the latter are used injudiciously, they frequently cause distress to the patient and delay symptom control.

THE NURSE'S ROLE

Although the prescribing of drugs falls entirely within the doctor's domain, the nurse still has a vital role to play. She has a responsibility to keep herself informed about the drugs which are available, about the way they work, their side-effects and contra-indications. Two heads are always better than one and there is no reason at all why an experienced nurse should not offer suggestions on medication when symptoms are proving difficult to relieve. She should also know the normal dosage of drugs. By referring back to the doctor any apparent discrepancy, she can help to eliminate the danger of human error.

Another important role of the nurse is in observing the patient's symptoms and the effectiveness of drugs. She is responsible for keeping careful records and reporting back to the doctor. Her basic training will have taught her which observations need reporting and acting upon immediately, but her constant surveillance also enables her to present the doctor with a far more detailed picture of the patient's overall condition than he can elicit alone. She will observe any variation in symptoms in relation to the time of day, to eating, to movement, to receiving visitors or to the administration of drugs, for example.

Apart from being well-informed and observant, the nurse is also responsible for communication with patients on all aspects of drug-therapy. She must be able to explain why certain drugs are prescribed, why changes are made and what, if any, side-effects can be be expected, and, in some cases, reported to the doctor. The accurate and punctual administration of drugs is also part of a nurse's basic training, but many hospital nurses fail to recognise their role in preparing patients to take over this responsibility after their discharge.

DRUG COMPLIANCE

There is little virtue in prescribing the most effective medication if no steps are taken to ensure drug compliance by the patient. Because of the wide range of possible symptoms, it is frequently necessary to use several different drugs, making compliance even more important and even more difficult.

Before discharge from hospital, every patient who is capable of doing so should have administered his own drugs for at least twenty-four hours, under the supervision of the nursing staff. The elderly, those who live alone, or the apparently less intelligent patients, should be given two or three days to become proficient and confident. On being discharged home, the patient should receive a daily drug regime chart. On this chart will be a list of times at which medication should be taken, usually beginning with '6.00 a.m. or on waking' and ending with '10.00 p.m. or bedtime if earlier'. Against each time is a list of the drugs to be taken, with the quantity and appearance, and an indication of what they are for. For example:

10.00 a.m.

Morphine Sulph.	10ml	Clear solution	For pain
Cyclizine	50mg	One white tablet	For sickness
Dorbanex	15ml	Orange syrup	For constipation
Prednisolone	5mg	One pink tablet; dissolve in water; take with milk.	To improve appetite

All instructions must be written very clearly, preferably in pencil, so that doses can be changed legibly. Whenever possible, a friend or neighbour should also be instructed. Drugs required o.d., b.d., t.d.s., q.d.s. or nocte are, of course, given at the most appropriate time on the four-hourly schedule. If analgesics are not needed, every attempt is made to reduce the drug times to twice or three times a day.

The strength of tablets can vary, e.g. amitriptyline 50mg could be dispensed as one 50mg tablet or two 25mg tablets. It is, therefore, essential that a liaison or community sister checks a new supply of drugs against the daily chart before they are used.

Drugs should be prescribed in as humane a way as possible. Diuretics need not be taken at 6.00 a.m., before the patient is up or properly awake. A nauseated patient should not have to swallow seven tablets and two mixtures at one time, whilst only having to manage two tablets at another. It is the nurse's job to inform and influence doctors in these aspects of their prescribing, and every doctor working with the terminally ill should have accompanied the nurses on a drug round at least three or four times. This is the only way that a true appreciation of the unpalatable size, quantity, taste and texture of the various pills and potions can be gained, plus the knowledge of which injections are painful or which suppositories irritate the rectal mucosa.

The following sections of this chapter outline those symptoms occurring most commonly in the terminally ill and some of the drugs which can be used to treat them.

ALIMENTARY TRACT SYMPTOMS (Excluding Oral Symptoms)

NAUSEA AND VOMITING

Nausea and vomiting occur in approximately one third of all terminal cancer patients, as well as in many dying from other diseases. The causes are numerous, but will mostly come under the headings of mechanical obstruction (tumour or impaction), electrolyte imbalance, drug-induced gastric infection, raised intracranial pressure, recent treatment with chemotherapy, or recent irradiation of large areas of the body. If untreated, the patient feels both exhausted and wretched. The cause of the vomiting should be established so that the most appropriate drug can be given. Anti-emetics fall into five main groups.

The Phenothiazines

The phenothiazines are often used because, in addition to their anti-emetic properties, they are invaluable as tranquillisers. When given with a narcotic, they will also potentiate the analgesic effect. For these reasons, the phenothiazines are often given routinely every four hours, either in a tablet or in a syrup which can be added to the morphine/diamorphine solution, or intramuscularly. Alternatively, they can be given eight hourly in a suppository.

The anti-emetic properties of the common phenothiazines are of equal strength, but their tranquillising potencies vary enormously. If the anti-emetic property alone is required, the usual choice is prochlorperazine (Stemetil) 5-12.5mg 4 hourly. When converting from oral to a parenteral administration, the dose remains the same, but when converting to suppositories, the twenty-four hour dose must be doubled. If tranqillising and analgesia potentiating properties are both required, the usual choice is chlorpromazine (Largactil) 10-50mg 4 hourly. If severe pain is present, methotrimeprazine (Nozinan) 25-50mg 4 hourly may be given. This drug not only potentiates the pain relief from the opiates, but possesses its own analgesic properties. Unfortunately, it is too sedative for many patients and is likely to cause postural hypotension, added to which, it is available only in injection form.

The emetic centres in the brain stem are stimulated by impulses from the alimentary tract, the cerebral cortex and the chemoreceptor trigger zone (CRTZ), which is closely related to the emetic centres. The phenothiazines act on the CRTZ, thus alleviating only that vomiting which was mediated by the chemoreceptors, such as narcotic drugs, digoxin or uraemia.

High doses of phenothiazines given over a longer period may produce parkinsonian symptoms, but these are amenable to the anticholinergic antiparkinsonion drugs. See page 154.)

Butyrophenone

Haloperidol (Serenace) is a butyrophenone, more commonly used in the treatment of psychiatric conditions, particularly paranoia and agitation. However, it has been found to be a most valuable anti-emetic in terminal care, being less sedative than any other. Since its action is on the CRTZ, it is particularly valuable in combating opiate-induced nausea. The usual dose is 0.5mg b.d. in capsule or liquid form. If parenteral use is necessary, it is a small, fairly painless injection. Doses of up to 1.5mg b.d. may be used, but this may produce extrapyramidal side-effects if taken over a long period.

Antihistamines

Although not all antihistamines have anti-emetic properties, several do. Their action is directly on the emetic centres in the medulla and they are, therefore, effective in all types of vomiting. This is thought to be due to their anti-cholinergic action. Examples of useful antihistamines and their dose rates are:
a) cyclizine hydrochloride (Valoid) 50mg 6-8 hourly,
b) promethazine theoclate (Avomine) 25mg 8 hourly,
c) dimenhydrinate (Dramamine) 50mg 4 hourly,
d) cinnarizine (Sturgeron) 15-30mg 6-8 hourly.

The last three drugs are particularly effective for motion sickness, but produce more drowsiness than cyclizine, which is the most effective drug in this group for the terminally ill. If given by injection, however, cyclizine causes a severe stinging sensation.

Metoclopramide

Metoclopramide (Primperan, Maxolon) is in a group on its own. It has a dual action, working on the CRTZ and the stomach wall. Peristalsis is increased, thus emptying the stomach contents more rapidly. When given parenterally, the local action on the stomach wall is lost. Metoclopramide causes minimal drowsiness and fewer side-effects than any other anti-emetic, but it can produce a tremor when combined with other anticholinergic drugs. To maximise its local effect on the stomach, it is usually prescribed before meals, 10mg t.d.s. in tablet or syrup form.

Anti-Cholinergic Drugs
Anti-cholinergic drugs, such as hyoscine, drastically reduce gut motility. Since its action is the very opposite to metoclopramide, the two drugs should never be used concurrently. Hyoscine can completely paralyse the gut and is, therefore, invaluable in controlling the vomiting of total bowel obstruction. It also has properties of sedation and the diminution of secretions, which confine its usefulness to the very terminal phase of an illness. The dose rate for hyoscine is 0.4-0.8mg 4-8 hourly.

When vomiting is protracted and unresponsive to an anti-emetic, combination therapy maybe necessary for a while. This may consist of prochlorperazine 5mg 4 hourly, cyclizine 50mg 8 hourly and metoclopramide 10mg t.d.s., half an hour before meals. Initially, it may be necessary to give the prochlorperazine by suppository and the cyclizine by injection. If long-term anti-emetic therapy is needed and oral drugs are not tolerated, suppositories should always be tried in order to protect the injection sites. If analgesia is also required, diamorphine can be given subcutaneously, or morphine in suppository form.

Once controlled, most vomiting can be prevented by one or two regular anti-emetics. There is, of course, no value in giving two of the same type.

Although nausea and vomiting are two of the most distressing of all symptoms, it is worth remembering that, in many cases of mechanical vomiting when there is no nausea, onlookers are frequently more distressed than the patient himself.

Hypercalcaemia is a common cause of vomiting in patients with bone metastases. The blood calcium can be lowered by prescribing either:
a) prednisolone 10mg t.d.s., reducing the dose to 5mg t.d.s. once the blood level is within normal limits, or
b) effervescent phosphate (Phosphate-Sandoz) tabs. i-ii t.d.s., but this can cause severe diarrhoea.

    If the level of calcium in the blood has become dangerously high, and more urgent treatment is needed, injections of
c) mithramycin (Mithracin) 1.5-2.5mg i.v. (depending on body weight) daily for a maximum of ten doses, or

d) calcitonin (Calsynar) 400i.u. s.c. or i.m. 8 hourly may be given
   initially.

In all cases of hypercalcaemia the fluid intake should be high and i.v.
fluids may be necessary.

CONSTIPATION

The problem of constipation is widespread in Western society, highly
refined convenience foods and a sedentary life being the main causes.
Amongst the terminally ill, the problem is magnified tenfold. The
constipating effect of opiates, low intake of bulk food, weak, lax
muscles, inactivity and paraplegia are but a few of the contributing
factors. The regular prescription of aperients will be essential in the
majority of cases. The correct dosage of any aperient varies widely
according to individual need.

Bulk Aperients
These act by increasing the bulk of faeces in the lumen of the bowel, by
absorbing water and swelling. In so doing, they stimulate the small and
large bowel to evacuate their bulky, softened contents. Examples of
these agents are as follows:
a) Lactulose (Duphalac) syrup is an effective aperient, but the large
   doses required and the oily sweetness of the preparation make it
   unacceptable to many patients, particularly those already nauseated.
   Made into a long drink with lime juice, a quarter of a teaspoonful of
   bicarbonate of soda and water, it is far more palatable.
b) Dioctyl sodium sulphosuccinate (Dioctyl Medo) 20mg tablets,
   (Dioctyl Forte) 100mg tablets – also available in syrup form.
c) Methylcellulose (Celevac) in 500mg tablets or granules. Cologel is
   methylcellulose in gel form, which many patients find easier to
   swallow.
d) Ispaghula husk (Isogel) granules.
e) Ispaghula husk, bicarbonate of soda plus citric acid (Fybogel) which
   is dissolved in water.

(c), (d) and (e) are particularly useful in the management of colostomies.

Lubricant Aperients
As their name implies, these act by lubricating the faeces. They are not
normally recommended for long-term use, as they have been found to
cause malabsorption and tumours of the mediastinal lymph nodes, but

they may be essential for patients who have used them habitually.
Examples are:
a) liquid paraffin,
b) paraffin emulsion.

Stimulant Aperients

These stimulate an increased rate of peristalsis in the bowel. Examples are:
a) sennoside B (Senokot) tablets, granules or syrup,
b) bisacodyl (Dulcolax) tablets.

Combined Aperients

The most useful type of aperient is one which combines a bulk softener with a bowel stimulant. Examples are:
a) danthron plus poloxamer (Dorbanex) as capsules or a syrup, the syrup being available in two strengths,
b) dioctyl sodium sulphosuccinate plus danthron (Normax) capsules.
Danthron causes a severe peri-anal skin reaction in some patients.

If the stimulant-type of aperient is given alone, it invariably results in painful colic, whilst the bulk softener given alone may result in a rectum loaded with soft faeces which the patient cannot evacuate.

High doses of opiates will certainly necessitate the use of aperients. A patient receiving oral diamorphine 30mg four hourly will probably need something in the region of Dorbanex Forte 15ml o.d., which should be given prophylactically rather than when the constipation occurs.

A sprinkling of bran on breakfast cereals, in soups, stews and in baking can reduce the need for aperients enormously. Although many older patients find this unpalatable because of its unfamiliarity, it is encouraging to see how many younger people eat bran and whole grain products. Approximately six dessert spoons full of bran a day should be recommended to those with severe constipation.

Some patients will require suppositories or enemas to keep their bowels functioning. The following are recommended examples of these:
a) Glycerine suppositories, which soften the stool and lubricate the bowel.
b) Anhydrous sodium acid phosphate plus sodium bicarbonate (Beogex) suppositories, which foam up, giving bulk to the stool.
c) Bisacodyl (Dulcolax) suppositories, which increase peristalsis in the lower bowel.

d) Normal saline enemas, which are the least uncomfortable, as they are non-irritant to the bowel.

e) Fletcher's phosphate enemas, which are disposable and therefore ideal for home use. Some patients with dyschezia can learn to administer these to themselves.

f) Glycerine enemas, which are made up of 100ml of glycerine and 400ml of tap water, are now given in preference to soap enemas. Their effectiveness is due to glycerine's hygroscopic property, which is less irritating and less potentially damaging to the rectal mucosa than soap.

g) Fletcher's arachis oil retention enemas, which are invaluable in cases of faecal impaction (see page 174).

h) Dorbanex enemas, which can be made up with 50ml of Dorbanex Forte plus 450ml of tap water for treatment of high impaction. Because of its two active ingredients, Dorbanex enemas both add bulk to the faeces and increase peristalsis.

INTESTINAL OBSTRUCTION

Intestinal obstruction is common in the terminal stage of abdominal malignancies. This is characterised by spurious diarrhoea, abdominal colic, audible borborygmi, and distension. When the obstruction is complete, the diarrhoea ceases and projectile vomiting begins. This is sometimes faeculant if the obstruction is low down in the bowel. Whilst there are bowel sounds to be heard, a bulk softener, such as Dioctyl Forte tabs. ii b.d., should be given plus an analgesic and an anti-emetic. If colic is still troublesome, diphenoxylate with atropine (Lomotil) may be helpful in calming down the gut motility. When bowel sounds cease and vomiting begins, a suitable regime is morphine suppositories 10-60mg 4 hourly and hyoscine 0.4-0.8mg i.m. 8 hourly.

In high obstruction, vomiting may be extremely difficult to control. Some patients prefer to have their stomach emptied by a naso-gastric tube. This may only be necessary once or twice, as a result of which the vomiting is often kept within tolerable limits for two or three weeks. The tube is, of course, removed immediately after the aspiration. Many patients remain on the verge of obstructing for several weeks and, even when it occurs, the lumen is frequently cleared again and bowel activity recommences for a few days. The stage of total bowel stasis sometimes last for three to four weeks.

DIARRHOEA

Though far less common a problem than constipation, diarrhoea may occur in patients with tumours of the bowel or following radiotherapy, chemotherapy, a reduction in opiates or the over-zealous use of aperients. The following are the main drugs that can be used:

a) Codeine phosphate 30-90mg t.d.s.

b) Diphenoxylate with atrophine (Lomotil) tabs. i-ii 6 hourly.

c) Mist. kaolin or mist. kaolin et morphine 10-20ml t.d.s., if the patient is not already taking an opiate. This is sometimes given after every bowel action, which is an excellent safeguard against prolonging its use unnecessarily or overdosing and causing rebound constipation.

d) Antibiotics or sulphonamides such as kanamycin, neomycin, phthalylsulphathiazole or succinylsulphathiazole, in cases of gastroenteritis. The appropriate drug would be chosen according to the sensitivity of the infecting organism.

e) Methylcellulose (Celevac or Cologel) for loose colostomy actions.

f) Patients with carcinoma of the head of the pancreas frequently suffer from steatorrhea, due to insufficient bile and pancreatic enzymes entering the bowel. The stools are clay-coloured, loose, bulky, very offensive, greasy and often difficult to flush away. Treatment with replacement enzymes, amylase, lipase and trypsinogen, plus ox bile in Cotazym B may increase fat absorption, reduce the bulk of the stool and reduce the frequency and urgency of defaecation. The tablets must be taken with food for maximum effect. The starting dose is two tablets with each meal, but this should be gradually increased until the stools become at least semi-formed and less frequent.

DYSPHAGIA

Dysphagia may be caused by pharyngeal candidosis (thrush), a bulbar palsy, carcinoma of the tonsils, oesophagus or larynx, or enlarged mediastinal lymph nodes. If candidosis is the causative factor, it may be treated with anti-fungal agents as described on page 135. Enlarged mediastinal lymph nodes are sometimes shrunk considerably by treatment with prednisolone 10mg t.d.s. or by radiotherapy. Where a tumour is blocking the oesophagus it may be appropriate for a surgeon to insert a celestin tube. Drugs have little to offer the patient with a bulbar palsy, though the overwhelming fear of choking may be eased by the use of an anxiolytic agent.

DYSPEPSIA AND FLATULENCE

Dyspepsia is no more common in the terminally ill than in any other group of patients, except for those treated with high doses of steroids or other anti-inflammatory drugs. It can be relieved, to some extent, if those drugs which may irritate the lining of the stomach are taken with milk or before meals. The following are some of the commonly used antacids:

a) Mist. magnesium trisilicate 5-10ml 4 hourly.
b) Aluminium hydroxide (Aludrox) 10ml or one tablet (to suck) 4 hourly, p.r.n.
c) Aluminium hydroxide and oxethazaine (Mucaine) 5-10ml 4 hourly. This combines an antacid, a local anaesthetic and a spasmolytic.
d) Aluminium hydroxide, dimethicone and sorbitol (Asilone). This combines an antacid and a carminative.
e) Cimetidine (Tagamet) 200mg t.d.s. and 400mg nocte. The inhibition of the production of hydrochloric acid will promote healing if peptic ulceration occurs.

Carminatives, which are substances such as dill, peppermint water, aniseed, gripe water, camomile tea and charcoal, aid the expulsion of gas from the stomach and intestines and are particularly useful in paraplegic patients, who are frequently troubled by flatulence. It may be necessary to pass flatus tubes daily for these patients, or even resort to the old-fashioned remedy of turpentine enemas to release the gas.

ANOREXIA

How often one is confronted with a patient suffering from severe pain and every other conceivable symptom, yet their only complaint is one of massive weight loss and poor appetite.

The only drugs likely to produce any worthwhile improvement in appetite are the glucocorticosteroids.

a) Prednisolone 5mg t.d.s. or q.d.s. A marked increase in the appetite can be seen in as little as forty-eight hours. The delight that this gives to both the patient and his relatives makes any mild side-effects which might be produced more than worthwhile. The mooning of the face usually improves the appearance of a cachectic patient. Ankle oedema may occur, but can be easily rectified by a diuretic.
b) Fencamfamin, thiamine, pyridoxine, cyanocobalamin and ascorbic acid (Reactivan). This is a useful 'pick-me-up' concoction, combining vitamins and a non-amphetamine stimulant. It is

commonly used in lymphoma cases where prolonged radical or palliative treatment has left the patient exhausted and anorexic. Its appetite-stimulating properties are sometimes quite impressive.
c) Bitters taken before meals, e.g. Dubonnet, bitter ale or sherry may produce a marginal improvement.

For a description of the nursing care of the anorexic patient, see page 168.

HICCOUGHS

Intractable hiccoughs are often seen in terminal illness due to uraemia or the irritation of the diaphragm by gastric distension. This can usually be relieved by one of the following:
a) Aluminium hydroxide, dimethicone and sorbitol (Asilone) 20ml stat and 10ml t.d.s.
b) Chlorpromazine (Largactil) 25mg stat, then 4 hourly p.r.n.
c) Methylphenidate (Ritalin) 10mg stat (an amphetamine-like stimulant).
d) Metoclopramide (Maxolon) 10mg stat, then 4 hourly p.r.n.
e) Warm vinegar 20ml.
f) A few drops of oil of peppermint on a sugar lump.

If the above treatments fail, metoclopramide or chlorpromazine are sometimes more effective when given i.v.

PROCTITIS

Proctitis is often troublesome to patients with tumours of the bowel, but it seems especially so following the formation of a palliative colostomy. A profuse discharge may occur and the anal sphincter, damaged by the tumour, is often unable to control its leakage. This excessive discharge of mucus can be very distressing to the patient who is already coping with a colostomy. Palliative radiotherapy may ease the situation or, alternatively, one of the following drugs may be used:
a) Prednisolone 5mg t.d.s.
b) Prednisolone retention enemas (Predsol) one enema p.r. nocte. These are best given at night with the foot of the bed elevated a little. Predsol suppositories are more convenient during the daytime.
c) Sulphasalazine (Salazopyrin) one 500mg suppository b.d. when the discharge is very offensive.

TENESMUS

Tenesmus, the constant urge to defaecate, is another common symptom following the formation of a palliative colostomy, when there is tumour left in the rectum. This is sometimes helped by treatment with chlorpromazine 12.5mg q.d.s. If there is coexistent pain, morphine sulphate will be more effective.

HAEMORRHOIDS

Haemorrhoids are a problem which occurs frequently, being largely due to the high incidence of constipation. Relief may be obtained from one of the following:
a) Benzyl benzoate, bismuth, resorcinol, Peru balsam and zinc oxide (Anusol) cream or suppositories.
b) Lignocaine, aluminium acetate, zinc oxide and hydrocortisone (Xyloproct) ointment.
c) Hydrocortisone, cinchocaine, framycetin (Proctosedyl) suppositories.

If the haemorrhoids are impossible to reduce, covering for ten minutes with a pad soaked in adrenaline 1:1000, followed by an ice pack, may be helpful. Rubber gloves or finger cots can be filled with water, their ends knotted, then frozen in the freezer compartment of a fridge to make leak-proof ice-packs.

ORAL SYMPTOMS

DRY MOUTH

Oral symptoms and mouthcare play such a major role in terminal illness that they are considered separately here, distinct from the other alimentary tract symptoms. Most patients become dehydrated during the last few days of life. When this is the end of a protracted and ultimately fatal illness, there is little or no place for the use of intravenous infusions. The only symptom of dehydration likely to cause the patient any distress is a dry mouth. This is relieved far more effectively by regular mouthcare, frequent sips of tea or drinks which stimulate the flow of saliva, as described on page 172, than by an infusion. The dry mouth is worsened in some patients by mouth breathing, by an inadequate dietary intake due to anorexia, or by certain drugs. The latter include many of the most useful drugs, such as the phenothiazines, tricyclic antidepressants and any other drugs with anticholinergic effects.

The following are some of the aids to effective mouthcare:

a) For routine mouthwashes, glycerine of thymol, peppermint, or glycerine and citric acid are all well-liked. A severely dehydrated patient, or one with obstructive vomiting, may appreciate having a jug of mouthwash and ice left at his bedside, to swill and gargle with as often as desired.

b) Effervescent ascorbic acid tablets also make an effective mouthwash for dry mouths. These appear to have the added bonus of reducing the incidence of oral thrush.

c) Glycerine, with its hygroscopic action, may be useful for keeping the tongue of a very ill patient moist. A pipette may be used to enable small amounts to be dropped on to the tongue.

d) Artificial saliva, consisting of methylcellulose 20, 12g, lemon essence soluble 0.2ml, and water to 600ml, is sometimes useful. This preparation is diluted with an equal volume of water before use.

e) Lanolin cream or soft paraffin are suitable for applying to dry, cracked lips.

DIRTY MOUTHS

Dry mouths rapidly become dirty mouths unless they are given constant attention. Teeth cleaning and mouth rinses should be performed meticulously. As always, independence should be encouraged for as long as possible and a mouthtray with forceps and gauze should be used only when the patient is no longer able to clean his own mouth. Hydrogen peroxide and sodium bicarbonate are effective in cleaning dirty mouths, but are very distasteful to the patient. If not cleaned properly, dirty mouths rapidly become infected and sore.

INFECTED AND SORE MOUTHS

It seems inevitable when caring for such grossly debilitated patients that some will contract oral candidosis (thrush). This is more likely to occur in those treated with steroids, antibiotics, chemotherapy or radiotherapy. It is possible to clean a sore mouth more gently by wearing a disposable glove and wrapping a piece of gauze around the index finger. This is dipped into the appropriate solution and gently swabbed around the mouth.

Patients with oral tumours, particularly following radiotherapy or surgery, may prefer to perform their own mouthcare. If the mucosa is too tender for this, irrigation with normal saline at body temperature may be possible, using a syringe with a quill attachment. If this is done regularly, it may be adequate to keep the mouth moist, remove debris and prevent halitosis. The following are some useful anti-fungal agents:

a) Hexetidine (Oraldene) is a useful antiseptic mouthwash for the prevention or treatment of thrush.

b) Nystatin (Nystan) suspension 1-2ml or one lozenge, administered every one to four hours. False teeth should be removed, cleaned and treated with nystatin each time the drops are administered.

c) Dentures may be left to soak in Milton overnight.

d) If treatment with nystatin is ineffective, miconazole (Daktarin) oral gel or amphotericin (Fungilin) lozenges or suspension may be tried.

e) Angular stomatitis is often difficult to heal, due to the presence of candidosis. Nystatin ointment is far more likely to be effective than vitamin supplements.

If mouths are sore from causes other than candidosis, the following may be useful:

a) Chlorhexidene (Hibitane) lozenges for sore mouths and throats.

b) Povidone-iodine 1% (Betadine) mouthwash for the treatment of all mouth infections.

c) Lignocaine (Xylocaine gel, viscous, ointment) relieves the pain of mouths badly ulcerated following chemotherapy.

d) A mucilage of lemon syrup 25%, chloroform water 25% and methylcellulose (0.5% solution) 50%, with soluble aspirin dissolved in it, is soothing in cases of oral tumours, or following radiotherapy to the mouth or throat, when the production of saliva may be reduced.

e) Mouthwashes containing folinic acid may be used following treatment with methotrexate. This drug is more likely to cause severe ulceration of the mucosa than most other cytotoxic drugs.

f) Carboxymethylcellulose (Orabase) for applying to ulcers and angular sores.

g) Hydrocortisone pellets (Corlan) provide the most rapid treatment for aphthous ulcers.

h) Triamcinolone acetoninide in emollient (Adcortyl in Orabase) combines a protective paste with a steroid.

i) Carbenoxolone (Bioral) is a substance derived from the liquorice root. It is thought to promote the healing of ulcers (peptic as well as aphthous) by increasing the production of mucus which protects the ulcers from enzymes.

j) Choline salicylate, cetalkonium chloride, alcohol, menthol and glycerine (Bonjela) is useful in the treatment of sore gums. These are frequently the result of friction from ill-fitting dentures. Since weight loss is so common in these patients, so are the latter. Many dentists will line the dentures in order to improve the fit.

SIALORRHOEA (EXCESSIVE SALIVATION)

This can be a distressing feature of oral tumours. Oesophageal tumours can produce a similar effect when the saliva cannot be swallowed. Mouthwashes of bitter ale or alum, and drops of atropine 2% may help to reduce the production of saliva. Tablets of atropine 0.6mg taken orally twice daily may also be useful. Barrier cream to protect the lips and chin, and a good supply of soft old linen for mopping up the saliva, are equally important.

RESPIRATORY SYMPTOMS

DYSPNOEA

The main causes of dyspnoea fall into six categories:

1) Loss of functioning lung tissue, due to tumour, infection, effusion, pulmonary embolism, lobectomy, or pneumonectomy.
2) Obstruction of air entry by tumours of the pharynx, larynx, thyroid or mediastinum.
3) Loss of lung elasticity, due to emphysema or post-radiation fibrosis.
4) Weakness of respiratory muscles in those with degenerative muscular diseases, quadriplegia or a high paraplegia.
5) Anaemia, causing an increased demand for oxygen.
6) Heart failure.

The respiratory rate is increased when the level of carbon dioxide in the blood rises, except in chronic lung disease, when decreased oxygen is the trigger. Opiates depress the sensitivity of the respiratory centre to the blood gases, hence their unsuitability in dyspnoeic patients with a curable disease. In terminal care, however, there is no other drug which can so effectively slow down the respiratory rate and relieve the anxiety which dyspnoea causes. The dose of oral morphine required will vary from patient to patient according to the degree of dyspnoea, but between 5 and 20mg four hourly is normally adequate. A great deal of breathlessness is avoided by those already receiving regular opiates for pain. Fear of shortening life prevents many doctors from adequately relieving dyspnoea in the dying. This seems indefensible when all that may be gained is a few more days of gasping for breath and overwhelming fear. The nurse who fails to challenge the doctor when a patient is left in this condition is equally guilty. She is responsible for reporting her observations and sharing her professional judgements.

If dyspnoea presents with bronchospasm before the final stage, a bronchodilator may be prescribed. Examples are as follows:

a) Salbutamol (Ventolin) 2-4mg t.d.s. or q.d.s. is usually effective. It is not advisable to prescribe inhalers in terminal illness unless the patient is already familiar with them.

b) Orciprenaline (Alupent) 20mg q.d.s.

c) Theophylline (Rona-Slophyllin) is a sustained release tablet, the usual dose being 125-250mg b.d.

d) Aminophylline 360mg suppositories given stat for bronchial asthma or routinely at night.

Tumours in the mediastinum are usually metastatic deposits in the lymph nodes from primaries in the bronchus or breast, or they may be the result of Hodgkin's disease or non-Hodgkin lymphomas invading the mediastinal nodes. A mass in this area may exert pressure on the oesophagus, the superior vena cava or the trachea and bronchi. The dyspnoea caused by this condition can sometimes be relieved by radiotherapy. Alternatively, glucocorticosteroids can be used and these are also useful in treating bronchospasm and lymphangitis carcinomatosa (the infiltration of the lymphatic system within the lungs). The usual choice is:

a) dexamethasone 4mg q.d.s., reducing to 2mg b.d., or

b) prednisolone 5-10mg t.d.s., reducing to 5mg b.d. This is a far less potent anti-inflammatory agent than dexamethasone, but may be adequate to relieve the asthma and chronic bronchitis which frequently precedes carcinoma of the bronchus, if this remains troublesome.

Pleural aspirations are usually painful and distressing, whilst the relief of dyspnoea which they provide is often short-lived. In most cases, a dying patient obtains far greater relief from the use of opiates.

Similarly in anaemia, 'air hunger' is relieved for so short a time by blood transfusions, whilst a small, regular dose of morphine can improve the situation permanently. Oxygen has only a very minor useful role to play in terminal care, unless a patient has long-standing confidence in it from previous illness. If it is administered, oxygen spectacles will be less distressing than a mask, but nurses must be vigilant to prevent forgetful patients from smoking.

If an infection is the cause of the dyspnoea, antibiotics may be appropriate, and if heart failure is the cause, digoxin and diuretics may be useful. Anxiolytic drugs, such as clobazam 10mg t.d.s. or diazepam 5mg t.d.s. will often be necessary, sometimes in addition to morphine.

CHEST PAIN

The pain caused by even the largest of tumours in the lung, with the exception of mesotheliomas, is usually remarkably mild, but chest infections are often painful. Once more, the opiates are the drugs of choice in the terminally ill. Repetitive treatment of chest infections with antibiotics frequently prolongs the process of dying in a quite inhumane manner, and for this reason is clearly bad medicine. This does not imply, however, that antibiotics should not be used earlier, when the expectation of life is still several months and there is a quality of life left which the patient finds acceptable. Even in those very close to death, antibiotics may make it possible to prolong life for a short period, which may mean a great deal to patients wishing to attend an important family occasion or to dispose of some important financial or legal matter. Four of the most commonly used broad spectrum antibiotics are:

a) amoxycillin (Amoxil) 250mg t.d.s.,
b) oxytetracycline (Terramycin) 250mg q.d.s.
c) co-trimoxazole (Septrin) (a sulphonamide plus trimethoprim),
d) chloramphenicol (Chloromycetin) 250-500mg q.d.s.

COUGH

Some coughs are dry and harsh, usually caused by the presence of a primary tumour in, or pressing on, the bronchus. Productive coughs are more common, usually associated with bronchitis, pneumonia, a lung abscess or an intrapulmonary primary or secondary growth. Treatment is divided into cough suppressants, expectorants, mucolytic agents and decongestants.

Cough Suppressants
These are mostly opiates, such as:
a) morphine or diamorphine, which can be prescribed in a syrup if this is found helpful.
b) linctus methadone,
c) linctus codeine.

Doses of the above vary widely according to the coexisting level of analgesia required.

Expectorants
a) diphenhydramine (Benylin) expectorant 10ml 4 hourly,
b) guaiphenesin (Robitussin) 5-10ml 4 hourly.

Both of these expectorants are most effective when diluted in a little hot water.

Mucolytic Agents
a) bromhexine (Bisolvon) in tablet and syrup form, 8mg t.d.s.,
b) carboxymethylcisteine (Mucodyne) 15ml or two capsules t.d.s.,
c) tincture of benzoin (Friar's Balsam) inhalation,
d) menthol crystals (Bengue's Balsam) inhalation,
e) menthol, cinnamon oil, pine oil, chlorbutol and terpineol (Karvol) capsules emptied onto a handkerchief and inhaled.

Decongestants
a) triprolidine, pseudoephedrine and codeine (Actifed Co.),
b) promethazine, ephedrine and codeine (Phensedyl).

The mucolytic agents liquefy tenacious sputum to facilitate expectoration. Steam inhalations are particularly effective. Expectorants stimulate the expulsion of sputum from the lungs whilst cough suppressants act on the cough centre in the medulla and also on the respiratory mucosa to inhibit coughing. The routine use of decongestants, mucolytic agents and expectorants is not appropriate when a patient has become weak and exhausted by months of coughing. It is sometimes useful to prescribe an expectorant and mucolytic agent in the morning, when the patient has enough energy to cough, whilst prescribing a suppressant in the evening to ensure an undisturbed night's sleep.

EXCESSIVE SECRETIONS IN THE LAST HOURS OF LIFE

Hyoscine (Scopolamine), 0.4-0.8mg i.m. 4-8 hourly, helps to dry up excessive secretions collecting in the trachea and the back of the throat. This will eliminate the sounds (usually referred to as the 'death rattle') which are so distressing to relatives and other patients. The use of suction for this purpose, although common practice, is very undignified and can cause great distress to both the patient and his relatives. If hyoscine is given for more than twenty-four hours, the dose will almost certainly need increasing to 0.6mg or 0.8mg, as tolerance develops rapidly. It is important not to give hyoscine before the terminal phase, as the side-effects of a dry mouth, urinary retention and a paralytic ileus will almost certainly occur. If given too late, when the lungs have already congested with fluid, it will be ineffective.

If a dying patient is in cardiac failure, so much fluid may suddenly collect in the lungs that hyoscine is inadequate. If this causes distress, the patient should be catheterised and given a diuretic intravenously. This is not a common occurrence, but it can be terrifying for a semiconscious patient and should, therefore, be treated urgently when it does happen. The usual choice of diuretic is frusemide (Lasix) 40-80mg i.v.

NEUROLOGICAL SYMPTOMS

FITS

There is always a possibility of fitting when primary or secondary cerebral tumours are present. These are more likely to occur when there are lesions in the motor area of the cerebral cortex or the temporal lobe. If fits are occurring frequently, phenytoin (Epanutin) 100mg b.d. or q.d.s. can be used prophylactically. This is an anticonvulsant which causes minimal sedation. Should this prove inadequate, phenobarbitone, 30-60mg b.d., can be given in conjunction. If lesion is in the temporal lobe, carbamazepine (Tegretol) 100-200mg q.d.s. may be a better choice. When a fit occurs and is prolonged, diazepam (Valium) 10mg i.m. stat may be given.

RAISED INTRACRANIAL PRESSURE

Cerebral tumours in any part of the brain are likely to result in raised intracranial pressure. Much of the pressure is caused by the area of inflammation and swelling around the tumour, which may damage a larger area of nervous tissue than the tumour itself.

The most common symptoms are headaches, vomiting (usually of a projectile nature without any feeling of nausea), diplopia or blurred vision, mental confusion and drowsiness. Other common symptoms, which vary according to the site of the tumour, are hemiplegia, dysphasia, dysarthria, loss of coordination, emotional lability and changes in personality. Most symptoms, but particularly vomiting and headaches, tend to be worse in the early morning when the patient has been lying down all night. Raising the head of the bed may help a little.

The inflammation and swelling around the lesion can be greatly reduced by the use of dexamethasone. As a result, the symptoms usually show a marked improvement and, in many cases, vanish completely. Since the tumour itself has not been affected, it will continue to grow and eventually the symptoms will recur. For this reason, the decision about whether or not to treat with dexamethasone should be considered with great care. Whenever possible, the patient or his family or both, should be involved. Since the improvement can be so dramatic, it is essential that the family and friends understand what is happening and that the temporary nature of the improvement is explained. So often, relatives are convinced that the patient is getting better. If the tumour is growing very rapidly or the patient is elderly or already comatosed, the use of dexamethasone would probably be inappropriate. If the patient is young and still has an apparent prognosis of several months, the improvement in the quality of the remaining life may make treatment very worthwhile.

It will be necessary to prescribe a high dose initially, dexamethasone 4mg q.d.s. This should then be reduced gradually to a maintenance dose of 2mg b.d., unless the symptoms recur at a higher level. Although long-term side-effects of steroids need not concern those prescribing for the terminally ill, the short-term ones must be considered. A ferocious appetite, obesity, mooning of the face, and psychological changes ranging from a mild euphoria to a full blown psychosis are the most common. If, in order to prevent the recurrence of symptoms, the dose has to be kept at such a high level that these side-effects are unavoidable, a gradual withdrawal of the drug should be considered when the next symptoms occur. Continuous short-lived resurrections of the patient, achieved by constant increases in the dosage, are inhumane and unethical.

If, after four days, the dexamethasone has brought about no improvement, it should be gradually reduced and discontinued.

The correct use of dexamethasone need not lead to difficult ethical decisions or a prolongation of the process of dying. It can improve the quality of life enormously; when the tumour has grown sufficiently to cause a recurrence of the symptoms, withdrawal of the drug can ensure a fairly speedy and peaceful death. As the dexamethasone is withdrawn, diamorphine and diazepam should be introduced to control headaches and prevent fitting. An anti-emetic, probably cyclizine, may also be required.

GENITO-URINARY SYMPTOMS

URINARY INCONTINENCE

This is a common symptom of terminal illness, usually caused by gross weakness and clouding of consciousness in the last days of life. However, it may also occur at an earlier stage, when the patient is fully alert and often distraught by loss of control and dignity. It seems to be the symptom which many patients fear above all else. The main causes of incontinence occurring at an earlier stage are damage to the bladder, caused by pelvic malignancies, prostatic hypertrophy, cerebral or spinal tumours, nerve blocks, too heavy sedation, and urinary infections. Since it is often only a transient state, it should never be assumed that urinary incontinence is permanent and every attempt should be made to re-educate the bladder by offering urinals or commodes hourly.

Urinary Infection

If an infection is present, the micro-organisms must be identified and the appropriate treatment given. The following are frequently recommended:

a) Nitrofurantoin (Furadantin) 100mg q.d.s., taken after meals as it is a gastric irritant.
b) Nalidixic acid (Negram) 1g q.d.s.
c) Co-trimoxazole (Septrin) tabs. ii b.d. (also available in soluble form and in suspension). Many organisms infecting the urinary tract are sensitive to Septrin. For this reason, in terminal illness where immediate symptom control is of paramount importance, it is not unreasonable to start a course of treatment as soon as a specimen has been taken, that is, before the organism has been identified.

Reduced Bladder Tone
If the bladder tone is poor and frequency, urgency, stress incontinence or night-time incontinence are the problem, it is worthwhile trying either:
a) emepronium bromide (Cetiprin) 200mg t.d.s., or
b) flavoxate (Urispas) 200mg t.d.s. Both are antispasmodics, which are helpful for some patients, but disappointing for others. If there is no improvement, the drug should be discontinued and an anticholinergic agent tried, such as:
c) propantheline (Pro-Banthine) 15mg t.d.s. and 30mg nocte. If the symptoms still persist, a tricyclic antidepressant may help, such as
d) imipramine (Tofranil) 25mg t.d.s. and 50mg nocte.

Because some of the cells lining the female bladder are hormone-dependent, nocturia or nocturnal incontinence in some post-menopausal women is caused by an oestrogen deficiency. This may be treated with oestrogen 1mg daily.

Catheterisation
Catheterisation is frequently necessary, and although the long-term risks can once more be discounted, it should always be performed with a strict aseptic technique. In addition, a regime of antibacterial agents may be given to every patient who has a catheter in situ, to avoid the pain and misery of urinary infections in those already severely debilitated. The following is a suitable regime:

1) Septrin tabs. ii b.d. for forty-eight hours when the catheter is first inserted, and after each subsequent recatheterisation.

2) The continuous use of a prophylactic sulphonamide or a urinary antiseptic. Two examples are:
a) sulfametopyrazine (Kelfizine W) one effervescent tablet weekly,
b) hexamine hippurate (Hiprex) tabs. i (1g) b.d.

3) If the catheter shows signs of blocking, or the urine contains a lot of debris, regular bladder washouts should be performed using one of the following drugs:
a) Chlorhexidine (Hibitane) 1 in 5000 in water, which will need to be performed once or twice daily.
b) Normal saline bladder washouts, if there is no sign of infection.
c) Noxytiolin and amethocaine (Noxyflex) bladder instillations, one vial b.d. High cost prohibits this product from routine use, but when other bladder washouts are too painful, due to local inflammation,

the combination of antiseptic and local anaesthetic makes it a valuable alternative.

Catheterisation should never be approached in a casual manner. To have a tube inserted into the urethra is a frightening prospect for most people and to have a bag full of urine hanging constantly at one's side can feel degrading. (Leg-bags, covers and disguises of various types are available but are used all too rarely.) Patients should be given a clear explanation of the procedure and the need for it, and a day or two in which to mull it over. Incontinence pants and pads, or a urinary condom for males, should be offered as an alternative. Dribble bags are also extremely useful for bedbound males.

Where prostatic enlargement or distortion of the urethra or bladder make catheterisation difficult, diazepam 10mg given intravenously or orally before the procedure will be helpful, both for its muscle relaxant and tranquillising properties.

BLADDER SPASM AND INFLAMMATION

Bladder spasm is not at all uncommon in patients with indwelling urinary catheters and in those with bladder tumours. This is not only extremely painful, but it may cause profuse leakage around the catheter. The same drugs that were recommended for poor bladder tone in the previous section should be tried.

Phenazopyridine (Pyridium) 200mg t.d.s. is a soothing, anti-inflammatory drug for bladder and urethral pain. Patients will need to be warned that their urine will become bright orange.

URINARY RETENTION

Occasionally, urinary retention is caused by anticholinergic drugs such as hyoscine, cyclizine, propantheline, or one of the tricyclic anti-depressants such as amitriptyline. It is more often caused by prostatic hypertrophy or distortion of the bladder or urethra. It is essential that the person nursing a patient with urinary retention is calm and confident, since any exacerbation of anxiety will jeopardise all attempts at relieving it. Warm drinks, gentle pressure over the bladder, running water, or helping weak male patients to stand up to use a bottle may help. Alternatively, one of the following drugs may be tried:
a) Diazepam 5-10mg with its anxiolytic and muscle relaxing properties may be useful.

b) Mist. potassium citrate promotes diuresis.
c) Bethanechol (Myotonine) 10mg t.d.s. may be useful, but its overall effect makes it unacceptable to many patients.
d) Phenoxybenzamine (Dibenyline) 10-30mg daily.

Urethral (or, occasionally, suprapubic) catheterisation is nearly always necessary.

VAGINITIS

The most common causes of vaginitis in women who are terminally ill are carcinoma of the cervix, producing a constant discharge, carcinoma of the vagina or vulva, a recto-vaginal or vesico-vaginal fistula, or candidosis. In cases of non-specific, monilial or bacterial vaginitis, rapid relief of soreness and lessening of discharge can sometimes be achieved by the use of one of the following treatments:
a) Hydrargraphen (Penotrane) pessaries 1.5mg or 5mg i-ii b.d.
b) Nystatin (Nystan) pessaries i-ii b.d.
c) Povidone-iodine (Betadine) douches. These are especially useful when fistulae or a heavy cervical discharge are present. The douche kits provided make it quite possible for patients to be taught to douche themselves. They may do this as often as four hourly for maximum comfort. If vaginal douches are too painful, jug douches and perineal wash downs may be performed with Betadine.
d) Yoghurt inserted into the vagina with an applicator is very soothing. In addition, it alters the pH, thus reducing infection and odours.

SKIN SYMPTOMS

PRESSURE SORES

Pressure sores are traditionally one of the greatest sources of guilt and shame for nurses. It is now widely appreciated that the damage which causes deep, necrotic ulcers has occurred long before the surface skin over the area breaks down. The tissue immediately covering the bony prominence is the first to suffer from the prolonged obstruction of its blood supply. Once necrosis has occurred here, it is only a matter of time before the surface tissues are affected. By the time the district nurse is asked to visit or admission to hospital is arranged, irreversible damage may have already occurred. The following are some useful preparations:
a) Arachis oil and methylated spirit 1:1, for gentle massaging of intact pressure areas.

b) Povidone-iodine (Betadine) aerosol spray for treating superficial sores.

c) Neomycin, zinc bacitracin and amino acids as a powder (Cicatrin) or neomycin, polymixin and zinc bacitracin (Polybactrin) for treatment of superficial, infected sores.

d) Gentian violet, useful for drying moist sores.

Treatments (b) and (d) are both impracticable for home use unless disposable pads or sheets are used, because of staining.

e) Chlorhexidene, aqueous (Hibitane) 1:1000 for cleaning open sores.

f) Edinburgh University solution of lime (eusol) for cleaning 'dirty' sores.

g) Hydrogen peroxide for desloughing 'dirty' sores (always followed by normal saline).

h) Malic acid, benzoic acid, salicylic acid and propylene glycol (Aserbine or Malatex) cream for application to necrosed areas to aid desloughing (this should never be applied to healthy tissue).

i) Hydrocortisone, neomycin palmitate, trypsin and chymotrypsin (Chymacort). By its triple action, inflammation is reduced, infection is controlled and dead tissue is desloughed by the proteolytic activity of the enzyme.

j) Bupivacaine 0.5% or topical lignocaine 4% are local anaesthetics which can be used for packing deep painful sores.

k) Ascorbic acid (Redoxon effervescent) 2g o.d. will promote healing in some patients.

The vast array of products available emphasises the fact that none is the panacea of treatment. It is important that the minimum number of agents is used, and that all staff act uniformly in the preparations they select, in order to avoid the possibility of interactions between different chemicals which may cause unwanted skin reactions. (For the prevention of pressure sores, see pages 163–4.)

SORE SKIN

Skin may become sore from incontinence, discharges, an overactive colostomy or ileostomy, or from dryness which is common in the dehydrated or anorexic patient. The following are some useful preparations; the skin must always be cleaned and dried thoroughly before they are applied:

a) Barrier creams, e.g. Conotrane, Siopel, Thovaline, or more simple substances such as zinc and castor oil or soft paraffin are essential for incontinent patients.

b) Arachis oil (Oilatum) as a cream or an emollient for using in bath water for dry skin conditions.

c) Lanolin cream for dry skin.

d) Benzalkonium and cetrimide (Drapolene) cream for ammonia burns caused by urinary incontinence.

e) Triamcinolone, nystatin, neomycin and gramicidin (Tri-Adcortyl) cream can be used when inflammatory dermatoses are exacerbated by fungal or bacterial infection.

f) Morhulin cream and powder, containing cod liver oil, zinc oxide, cetrimide and Dakin's solution, is valuable in the treatment of excoriated skin.

g) Carboxymethylcellulose (Orabase) is a thick paste which can be spread over areas of skin exposed to enzymes. This may be around ileostomies or fistulae tracking out to the skin from any part of the gut, or around any discharging wound.

FUNGATING TUMOURS

Many cancers, including those of the vulva, bladder and rectum, occasionally fungate onto the surface of the skin, but none do so as frequently as cancer of the breast. Radiotherapy can often help to shrink and dry the tumour, but many will continue to require skilled nursing care. Much can be done to keep the lesions comfortable and odourless, but the attitude with which the dressing is performed will do far more to alleviate the patient's feelings of shame, disgust and alienation than any of the following potions.

a) Chymacort, Malatex or Aserbine for desloughing.

b) Half-strength eusol or hydrogen peroxide for cleaning 'dirty' lesions (followed by normal saline).

c) Aqueous chlorhexidine 1:1000 or povidone-iodine solution for cleaning sensitive lesions.

d) Half-strength eusol and liquid paraffin for packing.

e) Yoghurt may be used for packing or covering offensive lesions. This maintains a pH in which most pathogenic bacteria cannot breed, and is also very soothing. Any bactericidal agents used to clean the lesion should be rinsed away with saline before the yoghurt is applied, otherwise the bacteria in the yoghurt will be destroyed and its value lost.

f) Any lesion which is inflamed and has an offensive smell is almost certain to be infected by anaerobic bacteria. Systemic treatment with metronidazole (Flagyl) 200mg 8 hourly is often effective in penetrating necrotic tissue.

g) Pads soaked in adrenaline 1:1000 may be useful when capillary bleeding is persistent.

h) Swabs soaked in local anaesthetics, lignocaine 4% or bupivocaine 0.5% may be necessary.

SKIN IRRITATIONS

Many skin irritations are caused by dry skin. These are best treated with one of the following simple preparations:

a) Arachis oil (Oilatum) cream and bath emollient.

b) Ung. emulsificans for washing, instead of using soap.

c) Lanolin cream.

If rashes or irritations persist, the cause will frequently be a drug allergy. Withdrawal of the drug may have to be undertaken gradually. Meanwhile, systemic antihistamines such as:

a) chlorpheniramine maleate (Piriton) 4mg q.d.s., or

b) promethazine hydrochloride (Vallergan) 10mg t.d.s. may be useful.

If the irritation is due to a chronic complaint, such as psoriasis or dermatitis, a topical steroid preparation such as:

a) hydrocortisone cream 0.5%, 1% or 2.5%, or

b) clobetasol propionate 0.05% (Dermovate) cream may be required.

Patients with obstructive jaundice frequently suffer from the most extreme form of pruritis. Bile, unable to enter the bowel, re-enters the blood stream and crystallised bile salts are deposited in the skin. This may be alleviated by one of the following preparations:

a) Cucumbers, liquidised and applied to the skin three times daily, will eliminate the itch of almost all jaundiced patients. It has no side-effects.

b) Cholestyramine (Questran) 1-2 sachets o.d. binds bile acids in the bowel, preventing their absorption and thereby relieving the itching. This is ineffective when biliary obstruction is complete. Maximum effect is not achieved for two weeks.

c) Crotamiton 10% (Eurax) lotion and cream, applied as necessary to relieve itching.

d) Phenobarbitone 30-60mg t.d.s. helps to detoxinate the blood by increasing the production of hepatic glucuronyl transferase, the enzyme that conjugates bilirubin and increases the bile flow.

e) Methyltestosterone may be effective, but may worsen the jaundice.

MISCELLANEOUS PHYSICAL SYMPTOMS

URAEMIA

Many patients become uraemic when they are dying. As a result, they become confused, restless and agitated with twitching of the muscles and hiccoughs. With the exception of hiccoughs (see page 133) these symptoms are usually relieved by:
a) diazepam 10mg i.m. 4 hourly, or
b) chlorpromazine 25-50mg i.m. or p.r. 4 hourly, or
c) hyoscine 0.4mg i.m. 8 hourly.

DIABETES

Apart from the number of diabetics found in every section of the community, two additional groups will be found amongst the terminally ill. These are patients who develop diabetes mellitus as a result of carcinoma of the pancreas or after treatment with steroids, as well as those who develop diabetes insipidus as a result of a pituitary tumour or following a hypophysectomy. The first group, those with diabetes mellitus, may need insulin therapy, but oral hypoglycaemic drugs are adequate in the majority of cases.

a) Glibenclamide (Euglucon) 2.5-10mg o.d.,
b) Metformin (Glucophage) 850mg b.d.

The second group, those with diabetes insipidus, usually require treatment with one the following:
a) Desmopressin (DDAVP), a synthetic form of the antidiuretic hormone which is given by injection or in nose drops (it is digested if swallowed).
b) Chorpropramide (Diabinese) 100-375mg o.d.

MALODOURS

People still talk occasionally about a 'cancer smell', linking cancer with the inevitable smell of putrid flesh. Few symptoms cause patients greater mental anguish or a greater feeling of isolation than the foul odours of some forms of cancer. Recto-vaginal fistulae, fungating lesions, ileostomies, maxillary antrum tumours, and infected, gangrenous pressure sores are just a few of them. It is one of the greatest challenges to the empathy, patience and ingenuity of those caring for patients with terminal malignant disease.

Halitosis may be a problem in patients who are anorexic or dehydrated, but it is likely to be far more severe in those with tumours in the mouth, pharynx, nose or nasal sinuses, those with lung abscesses or those with bowel obstruction. Regular mouthcare is vital.

The following are some of the substances which may be useful in combating these and other odours:

a) Glycerine of thymol or Oraldene mouthwashes and toothpaste, used regularly, will go a long way towards eliminating halitosis.
b) Sucking strong peppermints.
c) Chewing parsley is a most effective treatment.
d) Chlorophyll tablets (Amplex).
e) The majority of foul smells are caused by infection and are, therefore, often greatly improved by a course of systemic antibiotics.
f) Aromatic oils and essences (Nilodor and Dor) for sprinkling on dressing pads, bed linen and in ileostomy and colostomy bags.
g) Paraformaldehyde and carboxymethylcellulose (No-Roma) for use in colostomy and ileostomy bags.
h) Yoghurt (as described on page 148).

Other miscellaneous aids are charcoal dressing pads (Bandor), burning charcoal or jossticks, pine Airwicks, Cavalier fans with pine gels, aerosol air fresheners, extractor fans and the generous use of sweet-smelling soaps, talcum powders, deodorants and colognes.

Frequent use of soap and water, frequent changes of night clothes and bed linen, and frequent redressing of lesions will greatly improve the situation.

MUSCLE SPASM

Painful muscle spasm often occurs in paraplegic patients, those with tumours of the cerebellum and those with degenerative muscular diseases. It can usually be improved by regular passive movements (or active exercises when possible) and one of the following drugs:

a) Diazepam 2-5mg q.d.s.
b) Carisoprodol and paracetamol (Carisoma) tabs. i-ii t.d.s.
c) Baclofen (Lioresal) 5mg t.d.s. initially, increasing gradually to 20mg t.d.s.
d) Mephenesin (Myanesin) 1g 4 hourly.

HAEMORRHAGE

No symptom causes more alarm to patients and relatives than the sight of blood. This is largely due to the horrifying appearance of even the smallest quantity and its tendency to spread rapidly, looking far more than it really is. The use of one of the following may, therefore, do more for the patient's peace of mind than for his physical condition:

a) Adrenaline 1:1000 for topical use in persistent capillary bleeding.
b) Aminocaproic acid (Epsicapron), one sachet dissolved in water b.d. for haemorrhages into the bladder or uterus.
c) Menadiol sodium diphosphate (Synkavit). This synthetic form of vitamin K may be useful in cancer of the head of the pancreas or hepatomas, when obstructive jaundice leading to hypoprothrombinaemia is the cause of bleeding.

Radiotherapy can often be used to prevent the possibility of haemorrhage from superficial lesions.

WAX-BLOCKED EARS

Wax-blocked ears, although unrelated to the main disease, are typical of the symptoms which frequently distress the terminally ill. They must be treated as conscientiously as the most major symptoms, however trivial they may seem. Anything which makes communication difficult creates a far worse problem when a patient is anxious and in unfamiliar surroundings with unfamiliar voices. One of the following may be helpful:

a) Paradichlorobenzene, chlorbutol and turpentine oil (Cerumol) ear drops, applied warm, will take ten to thirty minutes to soften hard wax, prior to syringing.
b) Dioctyl sodium sulphosuccinate (Dioctyl) ear drops may need to be administered b.d. for two or three days, prior to syringing.

DRY EYES

Dry eyes are sometimes a problem when caring for unconscious patients with open eyes and those who sleep with their eyes open. Hypromellose 0.5% (Isopto Plain) eye drops are used as artificial tears. If the eyes are infected, they should be bathed with half-strength normal saline and treated with the appropriate antibiotic.

RENAL AND BILIARY COLIC

Renal and biliary colic occur occasionally when tumours of, or near, the gall bladder, the cystic or bile ducts, the kidney or ureter are present. Pressure on the ducts, dislodged segments of tumour, or stones may be the cause. The following are all anticholinergic drugs, hence their use in treating these symptoms by relaxing the smooth muscles:

a) Propantheline (Pro-Banthine) 15mg t.d.s. or 30mg i.m. stat. When given regularly, the side-effects – retention of urine, blurred vision, constipation and a dry mouth – are always problematic.

b) Hyoscine 0.4mg i.m. stat.

c) Atropine 0.5mg i.m. stat.

If the colic is very severe, it may also be necessary to prescribe a narcotic analgesic.

PSYCHOLOGICAL SYMPTOMS

ANXIETY

It would be a superhuman being who could live with the degeneration of his own body, endure the symptoms and treatments of a progressive disease, and accept the parting from loved ones and life itself, without ever experiencing anxiety. And yet, in any group of terminally ill patients, it is courage, dignity and cheerfulness which predominate. However, both apparent and underlying anxiety need recognition and treatment. The treatment of choice is people who care and people with time to listen. If communication with family, friends and caring staff were all that it should be, the need for anxiolytic drugs would be minimal. Drugs, such as the following, should always be used in addition to good communication and emotional support, and never as a substitute.

a) Diazepam (Valium) 2-10mg 4 hourly. This is the most commonly used of the benzodiazepine group of drugs. It is a tranquilliser with no troublesome side-effects. Given in the correct dosage, it relieves anxiety with minimal drowsiness, also acting as a muscle relaxant. A high dose will be effective in controlling agitated and aggressive behaviour, and is also valuable before distressing procedures such as reducing fractures, or a paracentesis abdominis.

b) Clobazam (Frisium) 10mg t.d.s. Clobazam 10mg is equipotent in its anxiolytic property to diazepam 5mg. This is one of the more recent benzodiazepines. Whilst producing the same anxiolytic effect as diazepam, it causes minimal sedation and muscle relaxation. It is particularly useful for patients who are still working and for those who drive, where any clouding of consciousness is especially undesirable.

c) Chlorpromazine (Largactil), promazine (Sparine) or trifluoperazine (Stelazine) are the phenothiazines most commonly used to treat anxiety. They are, of course, particularly useful in terminal care because of their anti-emetic and opiate-potentiating properties. Largactil 12.5-25mg 4 hourly is usually adequate, but acute psychotic incidences may require doses of 50-100mg. High doses can induce Parkinsonian symptoms, which may need to be treated with: (i) orphenadrine (Disipal) 50mg t.d.s., or (ii) benzhexol (Artane) 2-5mg o.d., rather than levadopa, the drug of choice for non-iatrogenic Parkinson's disease.

Some patients, especially the elderly or confused, become more anxious when given chlorpromazine. They may do better on promazine, but are more likely to respond well to a benzodiazepine. Unfortunately, this response cannot be predicted. Great care should be taken when drawing up injections of phenothiazines, because of the likelihood of skin reactions.

d) Haloperidol (Serenace) 0.5-1.5mg t.d.s. is useful in treating agitation, hyperactivity and paranoia, even when caused by cerebral tumours. It has a non-soporific calming effect.

DEPRESSION

Many terminally ill patients suffer from periods of depression. It will almost certainly be an exogenous depression, a healthy reaction to the situation, to be worked through with support rather than treated with drugs. However, the use of drugs is occasionally indicated when a depression is particularly severe or prolonged. This sometimes happens when there has been a history of depression, or when narcotic drugs have been taken over a long period of time. Some useful examples are given below:

a) Amitriptyline (Tryptizol) 25-100mg nocte. This is a tricyclic antidepressant, with side-effects of drowsiness, dry mouth, blurred vision, tremors and postural hypotension. If given in one night-time dose, day-time drowsiness will be minimised. It is essential that the ill and elderly begin on a low dose, gradually working up to the higher dose after several days. Premature increases invariably cause great distress to the patient. No improvement in mood should be expected for ten to fourteen days.

b) Dothiepin (Prothiaden) 25-100mg nocte, another tricyclic which is less toxic, thereby producing fewer side-effects.

c) Mianserin (Bolvidon) 10-30mg nocte is another useful tricyclic.

Interactions with other drugs and side-effects are minimal. In particular, its mouth-drying properties are far less than amitriptyline.
d) Nomifensine (Merital) 25-50mg t.d.s. Unlike the tricyclic antidepressants which only inhibit the re-uptake of seratonin and noradrenaline, nomifensine also has an effect on dopamine. For this reason it has a stimulating rather than a sedative effect, which is far more appropriate for many forms of depression, but which is obviously unsuitable for treating agitated depressions. Headache is a side-effect induced in about two per cent of patients treated with nomifensine.
e) Glucocorticosteroids (prednisolone 5mg t.d.s.) have been used in terminal illness for many years as a non-specific tonic. They produce a feeling of well-being and are often adequate to combat depression.

INSOMNIA

Insomnia is frequently the result of inadequate pain control, but may also be due to nocturia, anxiety or an unfamiliar and noisy environment if the patient is in hospital.

If pain is the cause, the evening dose of analgesic should be increased to one and a half or double the usual dose. If this is not effective, a middle-of-the-night dose should be given. In hospital, patients hardly wake up when given their 2.00 a.m. medication, and those at home should be advised to pour the medicine out ready and set their alarm clocks before settling down for the night.

Two other points should be considered before launching into the use of tranquillisers and hypnotics. Firstly, older people need less sleep and often sleep for quite short periods at a time, especially when they have 'cat-napped' all day. Secondly, there is little point in prescribing heavy sedation for a life-long insomniac, when he is quite accustomed to, and content with, his three or four hours of sleep each night. If a sedative is deemed necessary, one of the following will usually prove helpful:
a) Nitrazepam (Mogadon) tabs. i-ii nocte. This is a commonly prescribed tranquilliser of the benzodiazepine group. Some patients find that nitrazepam leaves them with a 'hangover' effect and they prefer, therefore, to take diazepam.
b) Dichloralphenazone (Welldorm) tabs. ii nocte.
c) Chloral hydrate (Noctec) syrup, 500mg-1g nocte.
d) Chloral glycerolate (Somnos) syrup, 500mg-1g nocte.

(b), (c) and (d) are three safe, mild hypnotics, especially valuable in treating the elderly.

e) Chlormethiazole edisylate (Heminevrin) 500mg-1g nocte. This drug has been found to be a most effective hypnotic in cases of confusion and agitation, particularly in those with senile dementia. It can also be used in the day-time management of this condition.

f) Promethazine (Phenergan) 25mg nocte. An antihistamine which is a useful night sedation for the elderly.

Barbiturates are synthesised from barbituric acid, and are drugs with hypnotic and sedative action. They are depressants of the central nervous system and should never be taken with alcohol, which potentiates their depressant action. Some of the more commonly prescribed barbiturates are listed below:

g) Amylobarbitone (Amytal) 50-200mg nocte.

h) Glutethimide (Doriden) 250-500mg nocte.

i) Phenobarbitone (Luminal) 30-60mg nocte.

j) Butobarbitone (Soneryl) 50-500mg nocte.

k) Quinalbarbitone (Seconal) 50-100mg nocte.

l) Pentobarbitone (Nembutal) 30-100mg nocte.

m) Amylobarbitone plus quinalbarbitone (Tuinal) 100-200mg nocte.

The barbiturates were once prescribed quite freely for insomnia. However, their addictive properties and the danger from overdosage is now better recognised and their use is ill-advised. In terminal care, their interactions with so many other drugs also create problems. Nevertheless, amongst the terminally ill there will be some patients whose general practitioners have been prescribing these drugs for them for years. Since the danger of addiction is not important in this situation, it would be quite wrong to discontinue their use if hospital admission occurs. With the regular use of adequate analgesia, plus tranquillisers if required, many patients will voluntarily give up their 'sleepers', but insistence on this would be inappropriate.

Alcohol is one of the most effective and palatable hypnotics. Taken in moderation, there are no side-effects. The combination of a warm, nourishing, milk drink with a drop of whisky or brandy is very acceptable to many patients with insomnia.

CONFUSION

The causes and general management of confusion are discussed on page 179. Drug treatment is mostly confined to the less sedating tranquillisers, as depression of the central nervous system will exacerbate confusional states. Examples are as follows:

a) Haloperidol (Serenace) 0.5-1.5mg t.d.s.
b) Clobazam (Frisium) 10mg t.d.s.
c) Chlormethiazole (Heminevrin) 500mg t.d.s. and/or 1g nocte.
d) Promazine (Sparine) 25-50mg t.d.s. and/or 50-100mg nocte.
e) Chlorpromazine (Largactil) 12.5mg at 8.00 a.m. and 12.00 noon, 25mg at 6.00 p.m. and/or 50mg nocte.
f) Thioridazine (Melleril) 25mg t.d.s. and/or 50mg nocte.

If the confusion occurs only at night-time, the prescription of a tranquilliser may only be necessary at 6.00 p.m. and 10.00 p.m.

More specific treatments of confusion may be called for on some occasions. These include the following:

g) The use of dexamethasone 0.5-4mg q.d.s. when the confusion is associated with a cerebral tumour. (See section on raised intracranial pressure, page 141.)
h) The reduction of any medication with sedative properties. If the use of opiates is thought to be causing the confusion, but these are essential for pain control, a cerebral stimulant, e.g. cocaine 5-20mg t.d.s. or dexamphetamine 5-10mg o.d. may counteract their sedative effect.
i) If the confusion is caused by the use of opiates in a patient already coping with cerebral atherosclerosis, a cerebral vasodilator, e.g. cyclandelate (Cyclospasmol) 400mg q.d.s. may help.

It is most unlikely that a confused terminally ill patient would cause harm either to himself or to anyone else. The latter would be the only justification for giving more potent tranquillisers by force.

REFERENCES

Baines, Mary, 'Control of Other Symptoms', in *The Management of Terminal Disease*, C. M. Saunders (ed.). Arnold, 1978.
Laurence, D. R. and Bennett, P. N., *Clinical Pharmacology*. Churchill-Livingstone, 1980.

Chapter 8

General Nursing Care

The intimacy which can develop between two people when one is incapacitated by illness and the other is attempting to meet his physical needs is rarely achieved in any other aspect of care. Such a high level of safety can be experienced when being blanket bathed, or having a dressing performed, that these are the times when the most painful questions are frequently asked and the deepest fears are shared. This places the nurse in a very privileged position, often making it far easier for her to provide the much needed emotional support than it is for the social worker or priest sitting politely at the bedside. The very fact that the nurse is busy 'doing something', and is not obviously giving intensive attention, makes it easier for some patients to talk openly, although others are inhibited by this kind of distraction and do need the undivided attention of someone sitting quietly beside them.

The enforced lowering of those barriers which usually prohibit physical contact, which occurs when one adult is being looked after by another, seems to enable many patients to abandon other defences that would normally prevent openness and intimacy. There are, of course, some people who find this obligatory physical contact very upsetting. In these cases, the normal conventions of personal privacy should be observed as far as possible, even when this means that some aspects of nursing care will be less than perfect.

The terminally ill are often emaciated, frequently bedridden for long periods due to weakness or paralysis, and are likely to suffer from a wide variety of symptoms, ranging from constipation to the overwhelming pain of nerve compression. Consequently, comfort is not something which can be achieved easily, and skilled, physical nursing care is of paramount importance.

HYGIENE

Hygiene in this context is not about high standards of clinical, antiseptic cleanliness, but is the word used to describe those personal tasks which are necessary to keep the human body comfortably clean and free of unpleasant smells.

BATHING

Bedbound patients will inevitably feel sticky and uncomfortable. Many forms of cancer, particularly the lymphomas, and several drugs, especially the opiates, cause excessive sweating in many patients. This may be worsened by the high level of heating in some hospitals, with which many patients are unfamiliar and uncomfortable. Some patients will be incontinent and some will have offensive discharges and lesions. It is not surprising, therefore, that the daily bath is one of the cornerstones of basic nursing care, and yet one frequently hears nurses proclaiming it to be an outdated concept. A weekly bath may well be adequate for a geriatric patient who is up and dressed, but a bedbound patient, particularly the terminally ill, will need a full wash of some kind every day.

There is no doubt that a bath can be a horrid experience. This will be the case when patients are told quite unexpectedly that they are to be bathed immediately, with no consultation and no time to prepare themselves, when the bathroom is draughty, the water is shallow and tepid, or when the patient is hauled about roughly in an attempt to complete the procedure in the shortest time possible. It can be similarly miserable for patients who are being blanket bathed, when they are left thoughtlessly exposed, when the curtains are left ajar, when nurses chatter together over their patients as though they are inanimate objects, and when the same two inches of lukewarm, scummy water are slopped about during the whole procedure. No wonder patients are heard pleading for one more day's reprieve, as though a bath were an unnecessary evil.

It can, of course, be managed quite differently. Patients should be offered a bath and, if a blanket bath, shower or strip wash are feasible alternatives, the patient should be allowed to make this choice. When people become weak and frail, they are often afraid of losing control of themselves and of their situation. Because mental and physical functioning have usually become slow and laborious, any attempt to hurry patients will cause them great distress. It is, therefore, essential to arrange a mutually agreeable bathtime in advance, allowing adequate time for the gathering together of thoughts as well as wash things.

When bathing patients, or indeed, when performing any nursing procedure, it is important to explain each step to the patient in advance. This is even more necessary when they are newly admitted to hospital, when a new procedure is being carried out or when the patient is confused or in pain.

As long as patients are able to climb out of bed and walk to the bathroom themselves they should be encouraged to do so, however much quicker it might be to bundle them into a wheelchair. The bathroom should be prepared before the patient is collected: the heating turned on, the windows closed and the bath run.

Even when too weak to stand, many patients get enormous pleasure from soaking in a warm bath. Hoists can be invaluable, particularly for heavier patients who feel more secure in them and who would otherwise worry about the strain their weight was putting on the nurses' backs. Patients who are in pain usually favour the type of hoist that has a firm seat to the less stable variety with canvas slings. However, some patients, especially those with spinal involvement, prefer to be lifted into the water manually when they are in hospital, if there are several willing helpers at hand. This can be managed quite easily by taking the patient to the bathroom on his bed. Two or three nurses can then slip their arms underneath the patient, all standing on the same side of the bed, lift him over to the bath and lower him gently into the water. Whilst he is being bathed, his bed can be stripped and remade, then covered with a polythene sheet and a bath towel. When the bath is finished, the patient is lifted back onto his bed in the same way. Once dried, he can be rolled onto his side while the towels and polythene sheeting are removed, then tucked comfortably into his freshly-made bed.

When blanket bathing patients, the water should be comfortably hot and strokes should be long and firm. When washing the arms, the limb can be supported on the nurse's forearm, as this is less tiring for the patient. When washing the legs, if the knees are bent and the soles of the feet placed on the bed, all the skin surfaces can be washed without effort by the patient or nurse. If time is allowed for soaking the hands and feet in the bowl of water, it is always much appreciated. The skin should be dried gently but thoroughly, especially where two skin surfaces are in contact.

Baths performed in such a way can be so soothing and relaxing that few patients will want to avoid them. It is the nurse's responsibility to create the conditions which make the daily bath a welcome luxury and not an unnecessary ordeal.

Baths are, of course, an excellent opportunity for the nurse to assess the patient's physical condition. Changes in the degree of mobility, the extent of oedema, or the development of pressure sores cannot be observed so clearly in any other manner. Dry skin can be treated with bath emollients and oil, hair can be easily washed, horny toe nails can be softened before cutting, fungating lesions can be showered, and offensive discharges can be dealt with. The daily bath is certainly not an outdated concept.

Frequent changes of night-clothes and bedding are essential, both for comfort and for the control of unpleasant odours. Garments of cotton, a wool and cotton mixture, linen or silk are far preferable to their synthetic counterparts, being much more absorbent and comfortable. Pressure sores are certainly aggravated by nylon sheets, pyjamas and nightdresses, and the latter may even be predisposing factors in the development of sores in the bedbound.

DISCHARGES AND SKIN CARE

The frequent redressing of discharging lesions, changing of colostomy bags or perineal padding are also necessary for comfort and for odour control. Colostomy bags can be applied to many types of sinuses, in order to prevent the skin from maceration and to reduce unpleasant smells. When changing the perineal padding of a patient with a recto-vaginal fistula, for example, it is not sufficient just to renew the pad. A thorough wash with soap and water (using a bidet if one is available and the patient is strong enough to stand), followed by a perineal wash down or vaginal douche, may be necessary three or four times daily. A barrier cream is then applied, the padding renewed and usually a clean pair of pants, nightdress and draw sheet will be needed. The demands which this type of care makes on a family, when no free laundry service is available, sometimes results in home care becoming impossible. If the standards are lowered, the skin may become sore, the patient uncomfortable and the house may rapidly become impregnated with an intolerable odour.

MOUTHCARE

Although mouthcare was discussed in detail in the previous chapter, a brief mention of the preventive measures necessary in hospitals to reduce the occurrence and spread of 'thrush' is called for here. The mouths of terminally ill patients should be examined thoroughly with a torch and spatula every other day. Any soreness should be reported to a doctor as soon as possible, so that the diagnosis can be confirmed and anti-fungal treatment commenced where necessary. All crockery and cutlery should be washed and sterilised after each use. Medicine pots left with traces of syrup in them are an ideal breeding ground for fungi. They need a thorough washing in hot, soapy water and, preferably, soaking in Milton for four hours. Feeding cups and beakers which are made of polythene and cannot be boiled should be treated in the same way. When a patient is known to have 'thrush', disposable crockery and cutlery should be used. Each patient should have his own wash bowl, mouthwash bowl and beaker (unless the latter two are disposable), and these should be washed carefully after each use. Face flannels and towels should never be left in contact with mouthwash beakers and bowls, as the former are another common breeding ground for fungi.

HAIRCARE

There are few ways of boosting the morale of a female patient more effectively than by a shampoo and set. Most healthy women experience a disproportionate sense of elation when their hair is newly washed, and this is equally true of those who are ill. In fact the pleasure seems to be magnified in many patients. Those high-minded folk who imagine such trivia to be meaningless to those who are soon to die are much mistaken. The ravages of illness can leave people feeling desperately unattractive at a time when they most need to feel confident and lovable, so that people will want to be close to them. If no hairdresser, friend or relative is available to perform this function, there is almost always a nurse to be found with a bent in this direction.

Some patients will have lost most or all of their hair as a result of cytotoxic drug therapy or irradiation of the head. Wigs can be provided by the National Health Service, but they may be a source of great embarrassment. Someone showing a special interest in styling and caring for the wig may well help the patient to feel more confident in wearing it.

Patients with spinal lesions, who are only free of pain when lying on their backs, can still have their regular 'hair do'. This is particularly straightforward when the patient is being nursed on a hospital bed. The bed-head is removed and the bed is then placed in front of the wash basin and adjusted to the same height. The bottom sheet is untucked and the patient can then be pulled up the bed on the sheet, until her head is over the basin. In this way, the spine is not moved at all. A second pair of hands may be needed to support the head during shampooing if flexion of the cervical spine causes pain. Patients at home will probably have to manage with one of the specially designed bowls.

MANICURES, PEDICURES AND FACIALS

Manicures, pedicures and facials are also greatly appreciated by a large number of patients, especially those who have never experienced such luxury before. Since few people normally indulge themselves to this extent, visitors will often be genuinely envious. This gives the patient an added boost, making a welcome change from sympathy. Volunteers who are willing and able to perform these services are usually scarce, but this situation is improving because the Red Cross are now running excellent, short courses to train more people. The Red Cross already provide a voluntary service in some hospitals and institutions.

PRESSURE AREA CARE

Factors which predispose to pressure sores are particularly numerous in the terminally ill. These include immobility due to pain, weakness or paralysis. Unrelieved pain will often make it possible for a patient to be comfortable in only one position. With paralysis, the patient may feel sore, but he is unable to move in order to relieve the pressure. Another possible cause is anaesthesia, especially relevant as a consequence of certain nerve blocks, when deep sores can develop of which the patient is totally unaware. Other factors which predispose to pressure sores are tumours of the bone or soft tissue, incontinence, discharges from the vagina or rectum, oedema and emaciation.

Vigorous preventive measures will need to be employed as soon as any of these factors are present. Beds should be kept free of creases and crumbs, and wet linen should be changed immediately. Frequent repositioning is the most vital single measure. Time spent explaining the need for this to patients and their relatives is time well spent, since few lay people have any understanding of what bedsores are, or how quickly they can develop.

To prevent superficial sores from occurring in patients who are severely emaciated and immobile may require hourly changes of position. If such frequent turning distresses the patient, it should be reduced to tolerable limits. In a patient with only a few days to live, dying with a superficial bedsore may well be preferable to the distress of frequent repositioning. No nursing procedure, however important, should be performed without consulting the individual patient.

Massaging pressure areas, the all-time number one preventative treatment, has been much disputed in recent years. Precarious, inflamed tissue can certainly be seriously damaged by indiscriminate rubbing. However, the gentle massage of intact, healthy pressure areas can be a means of ensuring that all sites are examined frequently, that pressure is relieved and that circulation is stimulated. In addition, patients find it extremely soothing. The sacrum, spine, shoulder blades, heels and elbows should all be treated at least four hourly in bedbound patients. A mixture of oil and spirit will not need vigorous rubbing in and does not leave the patient feeling sticky. When bed bathing patients, or soaping them in the bath tub, the opportunity can be taken for further gentle massage.

Dry skin is particularly at risk; the use of bath emollients instead of soap plus frequent massaging with oil or lanolin is necessary for a large number of patients. Oedematous tissue is similarly fragile and should not be rubbed. The careful manicuring of the nurse's finger nails and removal of rings and watches are vital factors in avoiding unnecessary damage.

Many aids are available to help relieve pressure. These seem to be even more necessary in hospital, partly because hospitalised patients tend to be more ill and partly because of the non-absorbent, hard nature of the beds. The first line of attack is usually the sheepskin undersheet, bootees and elbow muffs. Many patients find these hot and uncomfortable, however. Ripple beds and cushions are another great boon but are also rejected by some patients, who find them uncomfortable. Net beds have a limited use for those who already have large pressure sores but, psychologically, it is not often appropriate to nurse a dying patient suspended in mid-air. Split mattresses with sections that can be removed, foam blocks and turning beds also have a role in the treatment of deep ulcers, but the water bed seems to provide the speediest results with greatest ease for the patient. The vast array of products available merely emphasises the size of the problem.

Encouragement to eat a high protein diet and the addition of vitamin supplements may be effective in helping to prevent sores and promote healing, but would obviously be inappropriate for the critically ill.

POSITIONING AND MOVEMENT

POSITIONING IN BED

Careful positioning can make the difference between a patient who is restless, miserable and uncomfortable, and one who is peaceful and contented. An abundant supply of pillows of various shapes, sizes and degrees of firmness is an essential ingredient.

When a patient is nursed lying on his side, a firm pillow tucked into the small of the back will give extra support and prevent him from continually rolling backwards. A small, soft pillow, placed between the knees, and another under the lower shoulder, will help to relieve pressure.

If a patient is nursed prone for short periods, to assist the healing of pressure sores on the sacrum and hips, he will need only one pillow for the head (which is turned to one side), and one small one underneath each ankle, to prevent pressure on his toes. Some patients are more comfortable with a large pillow underneath their abdomen, so that the hips are flexed slightly.

When nursing patients in a semi-recumbent or an upright position, pillows may be arranged in an 'armchair' manner. If there is no back rest, this entails placing two or three pillows horizontally across the top of the bed (the lower ones are pulled away from the bed head a little, if the patient wishes to be semi-recumbent). Two more pillows are then placed vertically, one each side, to support the shoulders and arms. Finally, one more horizontal pillow is added across the top to support the head.

The value of adjustable hinged beds has already been mentioned in relation to pain control. They are also important, however, in the care of paralysed patients. When the upper half of the bed is elevated to bring the patient into a sitting position, his back, shoulders, neck and head are all still fully supported. This is not only more comfortable for the patient than conventional lifting plus the use of backrests and pillows, but it also allows a fuller expansion of the lungs; at the same time the abdomen is spared the compression which the otherwise inevitable slouching would cause. In addition, the elevation of the foot of the bed to treat oedematous legs, or of the head of the bed in cases of raised intracranial pressure, causes minimal disturbance to the patient. A further great advantage of the hinged bed is the lack of effort required from the relative or nurse. Patients can easily be 'sat up' single-handed, a great asset in home care.

It is difficult for a fit person to imagine just how intolerable the weight of bed covers can be to a weak, frail patient. They become even more hazardous when tucked in tightly. Many find it almost impossible to move about under the weight, some find breathing difficult, and others develop sores from the pressure and friction. The innovation of continental quilts is, therefore, a tremendous boon to patients as well as to the nurses, whose bedmaking time is substantially reduced. Where quilts are not available, bed cradles are essential. In colder weather, a winceyette sheet, at least, will be needed under the cradle, next to the patient.

Swollen limbs should be elevated for as much of the time as possible, either on pillows or in a sling. When patients are in bed, a roller towel and an infusion stand can be useful as an arm sling. If paralysis is causing external rotation of a leg, or foot drop, sand bags may be used with good effect. Even when long-term rehabilitation or recovery of the ability to walk is unlikely, any contracture or deformity should be avoided at all costs since it is likely to cause severe pain.

The provision of a 'monkey-pole' and pulley may help some patients to be more independent, particularly paraplegics with normal power in their upper limbs. Bed-sides may be necessary for patients who are restless, especially at night, if there appears to be any danger of them falling out of bed. These should always be lowered when there is someone at the bedside, and the reason for their use explained to both patient and relatives.

Bed-tables, adjustable to the right height, make eating, drinking and diversional therapy far easier to manage. Anticipation of the patients' needs, and the placing of drinks, tissues or newspapers within easy reach, will prevent the necessity of their making continual requests for help, which many patients find demoralising.

USE OF CHAIRS

Reclining chairs play an important role. The fact that the patient is able to sit out of bed gives a boost to the morale, while the weight of the head and trunk is supported in such a way that even the weakest patient will find it possible. In addition to the effect which this may have on morale, the weight of the body is distributed differently from when lying in bed, so that pressure points are protected. Dyspnoeic patients, especially those in cardiac failure, are often more comfortable with their legs down, and sometimes prefer sleeping in a reclining chair to a bed. The ankles, however, should be observed regularly for oedema.

Few terminally ill patients have the necessary 'spring' to get up from an ordinary easy chair, and the softer variety give inadequate support. Ideally, every patient should have a firm, high-backed armchair, with the seat approximately eighteen inches (45cm) from the ground. Ejector cushions are available for those who are still unable to get up, but these are not safe for the very weak, because they may be toppled right over. Footstools are extremely useful for swollen legs and feet, but should be used in conjunction with a sorbo ring or an air cushion under the sacrum, since elevating the feet causes extra pressure here.

MOVEMENT

Loss of mobility can be one of the most demoralising aspects of illness. In order to delay it for as long as possible, frequent, non-strenuous exercises will be necessary to maintain the maximum degree of activity, and consequently the maximum quality of life.

Where muscles are weak, the exercises used will involve active movements by the patient. These may be assisted, free or resisted, according to the strength of the muscles. The physiotherapist can teach the patient a full range of exercises, if he is in hospital, and he should be encouraged to practise them each day to prevent joint stiffness, to maintain muscle tone and to improve the circulation. In the community, this task may well fall to the nursing staff.

Walking is one of the best forms of gentle exercise. By improving the circulation, it has the added advantage of being one of the best means of preventing pressure sores from developing. Many patients are unable to walk unaided due to weak muscles, joint stiffness, lack of co-ordination, loss of postural tone and reflexes, or poor eyesight. These may be exacerbated by the fear of falling. Once confidence has been re-established, by walking first with the aid of two people, and then with one person, it may be possible to progress to the use of a walking frame, tripod or walking stick.

Terminally ill patients are often delighted by a positive approach to retaining or regaining their mobility. If such active treatment causes the patient distress, however, it should be discontinued, since the primary aim of treatment is the improvement of the quality of life. Pain, fractures or severe dyspnoea are three of the more common contra-indications to walking.

Patients who have paralysis of limbs, or who are unconscious, will need to have a full range of passive movements performed for them, at least twice a day. This entails flexion at each joint of the body several times, in every possible direction. The process will take about half an hour. It is essential that the joints are properly supported during movement and that undue pressure is not exerted upon them. Once again, the desired effect is to reduce the likelihood of joint stiffness and also to prevent the occurrence of painful muscle spasm and contractions. If the trouble is taken to teach relatives how to perform this function, it is likely to be carried out far more frequently and conscientiously than would normally be possible for the physiotherapist or nursing staff, in the more limited time at their disposal.

DIET AND FLUIDS

ANOREXIA

Although anorexia can be relieved in some patients by the use of anti-emetics or steroids, many are left with continuing weight loss and a very limited appetite. The nurse's response must be dictated solely by the patient's views and feelings, since many will no longer have any wish to overcome their anorexia, particularly if their life-expectancy is short, whilst others will demand great ingenuity and skill to help them to regain their appetite. Men seem to find it especially hard to tolerate a cachectic appearance or to accept any eating pattern other than three cooked meals a day.

There are five practical ways of supporting the patient who no longer wishes to be concerned with attempts to increase his nutritional intake.

One is the recognition of his wishes and acknowledgement of his right to decide what he will and will not eat, showing no compulsion to challenge, criticise or dissuade. It is important to appreciate that some patients, who might otherwise have lived for several months longer, stop eating in order to shorten their lives. They may feel that their situation is intolerable and see starvation as the only 'respectable' way out.

A second way of helping is to refrain from 'pushing' nourishing food or fluids at each mealtime, once it has been established that this is contrary to the patient's wishes. The nurse may well experience guilt in this situation, feeling that she is neglecting the patient, and she may feel angry with him because he has given up the fight for survival. However, these feelings must not be acted upon with the result that the patient is continually bullied to try to eat more, when what is really needed is 'permission' to stop struggling to eat. So great can be the relief, when this 'permission' is granted, that many of those who have dreaded the sight of food for weeks begin to fancy tit-bits of their favourite foods again.

A third means of helping is by discouraging relatives from force-feeding the patient. They are likely to experience guilt and anger in much the same way as the nurse, but these are often heightened at home, where relatives may devote many hours to preparing the patient's favourite dishes, which he then rejects untouched. If relatives can be encouraged to share these feelings and are gently helped to accept the inevitability of the death, they are more likely to find the courage to stop cooking and instead, just to be with the dying person. Every district nurse will recognise this problem and will have experienced the enormous tension that it can create in both the patient and the relative until it is resolved.

A fourth way of helping is by giving as little emphasis as possible to weight loss. Weighing dying patients who are emaciated and anorexic is insensitive and unnecessary. Scales are best kept out of sight to prevent their being a constant source of anxiety.

The fifth and final remedy is encouragement to buy a few new items of clothing. Nothing is a more painful reminder of the amount of weight lost than a pair of trousers three sizes too large.

The nursing management of those patients who are still anxious to regain their appetite and to gain weight is very different from that of the former group. It is important to provide a wide variety of food, served in small portions and made to look as attractive and appetising as possible. Patients frequently complain of being so 'overfaced' by a huge plateful of food that they cannot even try a little of it. Much of the food considered suitable for invalids, such as fish and milk puddings, is very insipid-looking. This, too, can be very off-putting, but a bit of imaginative garnishing can transform most dishes.

Another way of helping is to find out what foods the patient most enjoys and what time of day his appetite is at its best. Bland invalid foods are enough to destroy most people's appetite. Kippers, tripe, fish and chips or a good, hot curry are incredibly popular with very ill patients. Many of them are horrified by the sight of a bowl of porridge for their breakfast, preferring fried eggs, bacon, sausages and mushrooms, followed by toast and marmalade and a large mug of tea. This may be all that they want for the rest of the day, in which case they will need reassurance that this is very usual when someone is ill and that it is a perfectly acceptable pattern of eating.

Anorexic patients are often unable to face food which they have smelled cooking for any length of time before serving, and will soon feel nauseated if stale food smells are allowed to linger after meals. Good ventilation and well-sealed kitchen doors are very important. However, there are a few cooking smells which encourage the secretion of gastric juices, even in the most anorexic patients, such as the smell of bread baking or oranges and lemons being squeezed.

It is sometimes beneficial to use one of the proprietary feeding products to supplement the diet. Complan is an old favourite and can be added to porridge, scrambled eggs, soups or cheese sauces, for example, to boost the calorie intake, as well as being taken as a drink. Build Up and Clinifeed come in a variety of flavours and can also be drunk plain or used in ice-cream, jelly or sponge cake recipes, for example. Patients who find these products too sweet when prepared with milk may prefer them mixed with plain yoghurt. Hycal can be substituted for fruit juices and Casilan, which is ninety per cent protein, can be added to soups, milk shakes, fruit fools and instant whips, for example.

Naso-gastric and Intravenous Feeding

Patients dying on acute wards will frequently be fed naso-gastrically or intravenously, whereas for those nursed at home or in one of the hospice-type units these methods of feeding are extremely rare. The reasons for not feeding patients by one of these routes clearly outweigh those for doing so in the great majority of cases.

Patients find naso-gastric tubes undignified and extremely uncomfortable whilst intravenous infusions can be painful and they restrict mobility. Both methods are a source of great anxiety to many patients and they may form a barrier to the much needed, close, physical contact with relatives, since they too are often afraid of, and repulsed by, the sight of tubes and drips.

But perhaps the strongest reason of all for not feeding terminally-ill patients in this way is that it is rarely desirable or humane to prolong the dying process, once the terminal stage of a fatal illness has been reached.

Many doctors are becoming increasingly and understandably afraid of the possibility of lawsuits on grounds of negligence. To allow starvation to be a contributory cause of the patient's death is, therefore, seen by some as an unnecessary risk. It is also believed by many doctors that unpleasant symptoms will develop if feeding is not continued, even when the patient has lost consciousness. This is not found to be the case, however, and the prolongation of the dying process can in fact make the occurrence of distressing symptoms more likely.

Nevertheless, naso-gastric feeding may have a role to play for a very small number of terminally ill patients, at an earlier stage in their illness, in the treatment of anorexia. The regular intake of food will stimulate the appetite more effectively than any other treatment so if patients cannot tolerate food orally and are still anxious to fight on, naso-gastric feeding may offer the best solution. As always, this should only be done with the patient's agreement, not just as a result of pressure from relatives, or to make the medical and nursing staff feel better.

If naso-gastric feeding is to be used for a short period, the new fine-bore tubes will be a great improvement over the Ryle's tube. Instead of bolus feeding at two-hourly or three-hourly intervals, the tube is attached to a giving-set and the patient is 'drip-fed' with one of the proprietary whole food replacements. Feeding in this way can take place overnight, so that the patient is completely free during the day. The fine-bore tubes are less distressing to pass, less uncomfortable in situ and less unsightly than the Ryle's tube. In addition, drip-feeding has been found to cause less diarrhoea than bolus feeding. One added bonus of feeding anorexic patients naso-gastrically is that drugs can be given via the tube.

It is important to agree upon a time scale for this treatment, at the end of which the tube is removed, whether or not the appetite has returned. This will avoid the danger of prolonging the dying process and will also protect the medical staff from having to decide when it is appropriate to discontinue feeding. If the tube is left in until the patient becomes moribund, it will be far more difficult for patients and relatives to accept the discontinuation of feeding, and it will be far harder for the nurse who actually removes the tube, especially if the patient dies a day or two later.

DYSPHAGIA

Some patients are unable to swallow solid food, but get extremely hungry. The proprietary products such as Hycal, Complan, Clinifeed, Casilan and Build Up may be useful along with egg nogs and other milky drinks. The proprietary products are available in a variety of flavours and a choice should always be available. Naso-gastric feeding with a fine-bore tube may again be useful for a small number of patients who are unable to swallow because of a bulbar palsy or a head and neck cancer, for example. Once again, this will only be suitable at an earlier stage of the illness and then only if it is the patient's wish.

Liquidisers can be invaluable in preparing food at home for those who can manage puréed meals. Every patient has a different taste in food and a different problem with eating. Some patients with cancer of the oesophagus or tonsil will eat dry foods, such as toast, and clear fluids, but are unable to cope with the texture of milk puddings or porridge. Those with ulcerating tumours of the mouth may have to avoid any acidic items. Patients with oesophageal tubes in situ will need to avoid dry or sticky foods, and are well advised to follow each meal with a drink of soda water or ginger beer to clear the tube.

DEHYDRATION

Dehydrated patients, who are wanting thirst-quenching drinks to stimulate the flow of saliva, may enjoy fresh lemon, orange or grapefruit juice, peppermint or lime cordial, tonic or soda water, iced coffee or tea, beer and plenty of iced water. A dish of crushed ice and a teaspoon is all that many patients want. Chilled consommé and fruit jellies are very refreshing, as are chunks of fresh pineapple and acid drops. Regular mouth care, as described on pages 135 and 161, is essential.

PLANNING MEALS

The only essential ingredient in planning meals for such ill people is the patient's individual preference. This is one of the great advantages of home care. Relatives of in-patients should be encouraged to supplement the hospital diet with items of home cooking or the patient's favourite delicacies.

Although a well-balanced diet is desirable (and, whenever possible, one that is high in calories, protein and vitamins), the pleasure that food can bring to a dying patient is more important than the nourishment. Other important considerations, such as the appearance of food, the quantity and the variety, have already been discussed in the section on anorexia. (See page 169.)

SERVING MEALS

Immediately before meals are served, bed-bound patients should be offered bottles, bedpans, commodes, or help to walk to the lavatory, and a bowl of water to wash their hands, They will then need to be lifted up in their beds and made generally comfortable, with bed-tables placed for maximum convenience. Whenever possible, one course should be served at a time, so that hot food is really hot and patients are not put off by the sight of two or three courses sitting in front of them. Since the majority of patients resent the indignity of being fed, every effort should be made to enable them to maintain their independence. This can be done by cutting food up before it is presented, by the use of large-handled utensils, non-spill plates, feeding-cups for serving soup, and by providing adequate protection for clothing. Patients who are embarrassed by their own unsightly eating habits (those with oral tumours or a loss of co-ordination are particularly prone to this) should be offered privacy in which to eat their meals.

MANAGEMENT OF BOWELS

CONSTIPATION

The reasons why constipation is so common in these patients was discussed in the previous chapter. Since it is such a major problem in terminal care, the main causes are worth repeating. These are the use of opiates and related drugs, the low intake of bulk food, weak, lax muscles, inactivity and paraplegia. Apart from the use of aperients and a high fibre diet, patients known to be constipated should be consulted daily about their bowel actions and the information recorded. The traditional 'yes' or 'no' is not adequate in this instance. Some indication of the amount, consistency and frequency should be noted, and any bowel treatments recorded in the same place. A preprinted bowel chart for each patient is a useful way of ensuring that this information is updated regularly and is easily accessible.

NAME: Mrs X

REGULAR APERIENTS: Dorbanex Forte 10mls t.d.s. Commenced 15.12.82.

DATE	NUMBER OF BOWEL ACTIONS	CONSISTENCY	AMOUNT	RECTAL EXAMINATION	BOWEL TREATMENTS
12.12.82	1	Hard	Small	—	—
13.12.82	1	Hard	Small	—	—
14.12.82	0	—	—	—	—
15.12.82	0	—	—	—	—
16.12.82	0	—	—	—	—
17.12.82	3	Hard x 1 Normal x 2	Large	Rectum loaded with hard faeces	2 glycerine suppositories
18.12.82	0	—	—	—	—

After three days without any bowel action at all, a rectal examination should be performed. If the rectum is full, suppositories should be given. Glycerine suppositories should not be used when the contents of the rectum are soft.

When the rectum is found to be empty, but palpation of the abdomen reveals that the colon is loaded higher up, a small, disposable, phosphate enema should be given. In order to insert this above the blockage, a suction catheter with a wide bore may need to be attached to the nozzle of the enema. If the suppositories or enemas are necessary more than once, the aperient should be increased.

All patients detest bowel treatments, particularly enemas. They should, therefore, be avoided as far as possible, and nurses must take care never to underestimate these feelings.

FAECAL IMPACTION

Patients with faecal impaction are sadly not uncommon amongst the terminally ill. Treatment may take several days. The rectum is first emptied, either with suppositories or a phosphate enema. If the faeces are too large and hard to pass, a manual removal may be necessary. Since this may be distressing and painful, it is sometimes necessary to give diazepam 10mg i.v. before the procedure to relax the muscles and to induce sedation. Once the evacuation is completed, the patient is allowed to rest until evening, when 200ml of warm arachis oil are inserted as high into the colon as possible, with the foot of the bed elevated a few inches. There may be slight leakage overnight, so one or two incontinence sheets must be left in position. In the morning, a further rectal examination should be performed. If previous treatments have brought the softened contents of the colon down into the rectum, an enema consisting of one and a half pints of normal saline can be given. If the rectum is empty, a high enema of Dorbanex Forte may be required. It will be necessary to repeat the enema daily until a large result is obtained and no faecal mass can be felt on abdominal palpation. Aperients should have been commenced as soon as a diagnosis of impaction was made. Until these produce spontaneous bowel actions, suppositories should be given daily to prevent further impaction from developing.

THE PARAPLEGIC PATIENT

Patients with long-term paraplegia from an accident are often able to regulate spontaneous bowel actions with diet and aperients, knowing exactly when their bowels will open. Even if this is not achieved, almost all are able to perform manual removals or give themselves suppositories quite independently. The terminally ill patient who develops a paraplegia is usually different. He is generally weak and weary and rarely has the agility or the motivation to achieve this kind of independence. There are several different ways of dealing with this problem, the following being just one which has proved satisfactory for many patients. The contents of the lower bowel are allowed to become fairly firm, to reduce the risk of leakage or incontinence. If high doses of analgesia are being taken, a mild aperient may still be necessary. If the contents become too soft, a 30mg codeine phosphate tablet may be given on alternate days. Two suppositories, one glycerine and one Dulcolax, are given after breakfast every other day. Half an hour later, the patient is lifted onto a commode or lavatory. If a bowel action does not occur, the patient is lifted back onto the bed, placed in the left lateral position and a manual removal is performed. If the rectal examination, which should always precede the insertion of the suppositories, reveals an empty rectum, a high phosphate enema may be necessary.

FISTULAE

The care of a patient with a recto-vaginal fistula has already been described in the hygiene section of this chapter. If formed faeces are being passed per vagina, however, one additional possibility is the use of a tampon. This will help to reduce irritation and infection in the vagina and may help to prevent incontinence.

Recto-vesical fistulae can present an enormous problem with urine pouring constantly into the rectum. A urinary catheter may help, but drainage is often impossible due to gross infection of the bladder by bacteria from the bowel. The formation of an ileal conduit may be appropriate if the patient is fit enough, but the development of such a fistula in the terminal stage of an illness can only be managed by frequent washing and padding, with liberal use of barrier creams.

COLOSTOMIES AND ILEOSTOMIES

Colostomies are a common feature of terminal care, whilst ileostomies are seen just occasionally. Since the introduction of nurses specially trained in stoma care, the pre-operative and post-operative teaching and support of these patients has improved enormously. As a result, many terminally ill patients are able to continue looking after their own stomas almost until they die. Whilst such independence should be praised and encouraged, it does not mean that the nurse takes no responsibility at all. The skin around the stoma should be observed carefully. If any maceration occurs, it should be protected with a substance which will also promote healing, such as karaya gum or Stomahesive. The regularity and consistency of bowel actions should be recorded, and help may be needed in choosing an appropriate diet. A regular check should be kept on the patient's stock of appliances so that fresh supplies are re-ordered in good time. Most patients are taught to keep their colostomy bags on when bathing. However, if the motions are formed and regular, it is very beneficial for the skin around the stoma to be given a good soak occasionally.

Fear of colostomies and ileostomies prevents many people from offering to care for a relative at home. Nurses need to be sensitive to this, and they should be prepared to give time and attention to help families overcome their fears. The first step is to listen for as long as is necessary to the worries. The second is to give a clear, simple explanation of what a colostomy or ileostomy is and how it functions. Diagrams are essential. The third step is to encourage them to watch whilst a nurse, or the patient himself, changes the appliance. The last step is to support the relative to perform the task. A similar pattern can be used when teaching relatives to perform other procedures, such as dressings, or giving injections or suppositories. It is essential to remember that very little information is ever understood or retained if the associated fears are not dealt with first. The distress can form a complete block to comprehension, and the relative may appear stupid or uncaring.

INCONTINENCE

However carefully and skilfully bowel management is carried out, there will always be some patients who are incontinent of faeces. The cause may be residual or recurrent rectal tumour, or bowel control may have been damaged by a nerve block or rectal surgery. A few patients will have cerebral impairment, and some will have an atonic bowel as a result of gross weakness. It may be possible to manage these patients in the same way as paraplegics, but there are sure to be the occasional mishaps. When this happens, the attitude of the nurse towards the patient is of enormous importance, not only in her facial expression and in what she says, but in the way she handles the patient as she washes and changes him. No matter how reassuring her words are, if her manner is rough or hurried the patient will sense any disgust or disapproval, and his embarrassment and shame will be heightened.

Severely depressed patients will sometimes be incontinent for no apparent physical reason. It should never be assumed that this form of regression or attention seeking is under conscious control, and no blame or responsibility should be placed upon the patient. Of course it is unpleasant for the person who has to clean up someone who has been incontinent, but this is negligible when compared with the humiliation experienced by the patient. The person who cannot feel compassion for an incontinent patient should not be nursing the sick.

VOMITING

When a patient is vomiting, nurses sometimes have a tendency to rush around fetching excess vomit bowls and drawing up anti-emetics, whilst other aspects of care may be neglected. After the provision of a suitable receiver, the next most important factor is privacy, especially for those patients who are in hospital. Once the curtains are drawn, most people will welcome the comfort of a nurse sitting quietly and reassuringly beside them. When actually vomiting, an arm around the shoulders and a firm hand pressed against the forehead will not only feel comforting, but it will minimise any pain which may be induced by the retching, particularly if there are lesions in the spine. Used bowls should be removed as soon as the patient is well enough to be left for a moment, but they are better left covered at the bedside for a while rather than deserting the patient whilst he is still vomiting. If the patient has dentures, they should be removed and put in a safe place.

A refreshing mouthwash and a warm hands and face wash are usually much appreciated once the vomiting has subsided. At this point, an anti-emetic may be appropriate and, whenever time allows, the nurse should remain at the bedside until the patient begins to doze off to sleep. Night clothes or bedding which have been soiled should be changed at once to eliminate any residual smell.

FUNGATING TUMOURS

Some fungating tumours are small, crusty areas, which merely need to be kept clean and dry. A little protective padding may be necessary to prevent the clothing from rubbing and damaging the surface. Unfortunately, many fungating tumours are large moist areas, with deep ulceration, local infection, offensive exudate, and capillary bleeding. They may need daily or twice daily dressings.

If bleeding is a problem, it is advisable to remove the outer layers of the dressing and then help the patient into a warm bath. The inner layers will usually soak off easily in the water. When the bath is completed, a shower attachment can be used to clean the fungating area, so long as the water pressure is kept low. The lesion must then be cleaned using an aseptic technique. The solution used will vary according to the sensitivity and cleanliness of the area. A desloughing agent may be necessary (see page 148). A pad soaked in adrenaline may be applied if bleeding occurs, or one soaked in a local anaesthetic if the ulcerated areas are painful. Deep cavities are best packed with half-strength eusol and liquid paraffin to prevent infection and to promote granulation.

If the packing dries out and sticks before the next dressing is performed, one end of an intravenous cannula can be sited deep inside the cavity, whilst the other end is allowed to protrude through the dressing. Small quantities of eusol and liquid paraffin can then be injected with a syringe through the cannula into the pack, two or three times daily, thus keeping it moist and preventing sticking. Raw-looking surface areas can be covered with paraffin gauze. Gauze soaked in plain yoghurt may be placed on top of the paraffin gauze or, alternatively, Bandor pads, if offensive odours are a problem. It is important to discuss the effectiveness of deodorising agents with the patient, since their experience will be more acute and more constant than that of an observer. Several layers of padding may be necessary, and these are best kept in place with tubular elastic netting, to protect the skin from the damage of adhesive strapping which is being constantly removed and replaced.

DYSPNOEA

No symptom is more frightening to the patient and more distressing to his family than dyspnoea. To sit with someone fighting to breathe, whilst unable to do anything to help, is the terrible experience and haunting memory of many relatives. Remembering the high percentage of deaths from carcinoma of the bronchus and the many tumours which metastasise to the lungs, it is not surprising that dyspnoea rears its ugly head so often. It should always be remembered, when caring for dyspnoeic patients in hospital, that their panic and agitation may be the result of many long nights at home with no drugs or nurse on hand.

It will be necessary to spend a great deal of time rearranging pillows or lifting patients up in the bed, so that as upright a position as possible can be maintained in order to allow maximum expansion of the lungs. Some patients will prefer to be sitting in a chair most of the time, whilst those nursed in bed may be helped by a foot board or 'donkey' (a pillow wrapped in a draw-sheet which is tucked in under each side of the mattress) to prevent slipping down in the bed. Elevating the foot of the bed is also useful. Whenever possible, dyspnoeic patients should be nursed near to a window or door, to prevent feelings of suffocation and to alleviate fears of not being able to get any air. A cool, circulating atmosphere is essential, and in warm weather fans or air conditioning will be a great boon.

LYMPHOEDEMA

In addition to elevating swollen limbs, use can be made of compression pumps. These have boot and sleeve attachments which are pumped full of air, thus compressing the swollen limbs. The pressure can be regulated to meet the needs of the individual patient, and the pump can be used for varying periods of time, ranging from fifteen minutes daily to half an hour four times a day. Used in conjunction with diuretics, dramatic improvement is sometimes procured. Even if the size of the limb is not greatly reduced, the tissues often become far softer, and movement is less painful. Unfortunately, this is only likely to be the case if the lymphoedema is recent. If the symptom is long-standing, results are generally disappointing.

CONFUSIONAL STATES

Approximately fifty per cent of terminally ill patients experience some degree of confusion. For the great majority of these it is for a relatively short period at the very end of life when they are slipping into unconsciousness. However, a number of patients experience extreme confusion at an earlier stage in their illness, and for a longer time.

Confusional states fall into two categories, acute and chronic brain syndromes. The chronic syndrome is characterised by a diminution of brain function, due to damage of nerve tissue by cerebral tumours, cerebrovascular accidents, or senile dementia. There is no clouding of consciousness and the patient is labile, apathetic, has a severe loss of short-term memory, repeats the same tales of the past continuously and has inappropriate emotional responses. The acute confusional state or delirium has a reversible cause, such as a full bladder, constipation, unrelieved pain, biochemical imbalance, hypoxia from cardiac and respiratory failure, the patient's psychological state or the drugs which he is receiving. It always produces some clouding of consciousness and the patient is agitated. He may have hallucinations and delusions, he frequently misperceives and displays manifestations of psychotic behaviour.

Some confusional states can if their cause is known be relieved quite easily, and many of those which cannot be relieved are effectively treated with drugs. Those patients whose confusion cannot be cured are often greatly relieved by having the cause explained to them. Even confirmation of a brain tumour may seem less frightening than going mad.

Every attempt should be made to avoid humiliating the demented patient by exposing his loss of memory and disorientation. Information about where he is, who he is and what time of day it is, should be given frequently in the course of conversation. The use of night lights and the removal of any objects which might be misperceived and misinterpreted as something sinister can help greatly. Patients with dementia should be nursed at home whenever possible, since their confusion is sure to be heightened by an unfamiliar environment and routine, and by unfamiliar staff.

Delirious patients often become very uncooperative in their care and sometimes aggressive. Medication is frequently refused. Coaxing may be appropriate, but force is never so. Medical and nursing staff should think very carefully about which of the confused patient's nursing care and medication really is essential. Recognition of his right to refuse treatment, and some attempt to meet him half-way, may be all that is necessary. The confused patient at home, though refusing to cooperate with his family who are caring for him all the time, may be quite angelic with the district nurse. However, in hospital, patients are far more likely to cooperate if the help of a trusted and familiar visitor is enlisted, especially if there is any sign of paranoia.

It is generally not helpful to collude with a patient's confused thinking as if it were true, though there can be no hard and fast rules. One old lady of ninety-seven asked the nurses the same questions every day at frequent intervals. 'Have you heard anything of my dear Mama or my darling sister? I just cannot understand why none of my friends ever visit to bring me word of them. I worry about them terribly. Do you think it's something I've said or done which prevents any of my dear ones from coming to visit me?' Gently reminding her of her own age, and of the fact that all of her close friends and relations had died, seemed the right response when the questions were asked for the first time each day. However, no one could feel justified in repeating such a distressing response over and over again. Instead, the nurses listened attentively to her worries, telling her how sorry they were about her anxieties. Every attempt should be made to keep the patient as much in touch with reality as possible. An established daily routine, with regular meal times, bath times, visitors and bedtime, will increase the confused patient's feeling of security. Since making choices may be difficult, some decisions will have to be made on the patient's behalf, but this should be done with maximum tact and respect. People who are confused are as easily hurt as anyone else.

RESTLESSNESS

Relatives are often disturbed by a patient's restlessness which, like confusion, often occurs when patients are losing consciousness during the last days of life. This need not be regarded as inevitable and every effort should be made to discover the reason for it. Some of the more common causes are a full bladder, a loaded rectum, or pain. Catheterisation, a manual evacuation of faeces or increased analgesia should be tried accordingly.

If no obvious cause can be found, a tranquillising drug may be necessary, but this will not obviate the need for someone to sit at the bedside. Quiet conversation and the reassurance of a hand being held may have a very calming effect.

Bed-sides may be necessary to prevent falling, but they may need to be padded to prevent injuries. If bed-clothes are being continually kicked off, it is helpful to dress patients in pyjamas and cover them with a light-weight, cellular blanket which is not tucked in. This will keep them unrestricted, warm and respectable, whilst avoiding the frustration to both patient and nurse of constantly remaking the bed.

LAST OFFICES

After a patient has died in hospital, it is the nurse's role to perform the last offices, although patients dying at home are usually laid out by the undertaker nowadays, unless the nurse happens to be present at the time of death. Grieving relatives or friends should never be hurried away from the bedside, but should be encouraged and supported to stay with the body for a while, allowing the full impact of what has happened to start sinking in. Grief is likely to be expressed far more openly by people from almost any culture other than our own. This behaviour should never be discouraged, but the feelings of other patients and relatives must be considered. This may necessitate moving the body and the mourners right away from the ward area.

To help to eliminate fear of the dead body, the nurse should be seen to touch it, encouraging the relatives to do likewise. When the family are quite ready to leave the bedside, they should be taken somewhere quiet and private, with reassurance that they will be able to see the body again later, both in the hospital and later still at the undertaker's.

It is not uncommon for nurses to be seen performing last offices in an indifferent or giggly manner, but both these forms of behaviour are defence mechanisms. Although they may appear insensitive and uncaring, this type of response is inevitable when there is no facility for the nurses to obtain support and deal adequately with their own feelings about death. Relatives can be caused a great deal of unnecessary pain if they are unfortunate enough to witness such inappropriate behaviour. Ideally, the nurse's manner at this time should be quiet and respectful. More senior staff should be sensitive to the turmoil of emotion which their juniors are experiencing, and should encourage them to share their feelings, be they shock, fear, repulsion or sadness. Given the right kind of support, there is frequently an outburst of anger at the cruelty of death, particularly if the deceased was still young, in which case the junior nurse might be identifying strongly with them.

Every effort should be made to prevent the appearance of the body from causing distress to the family. The dentures should be replaced and the jaw closed securely. If the eyelids of an emaciated patient are difficult to keep closed, a piece of adhesive tape, such as Micropore, can be used temporarily. A corpse with mouth or eyes open makes a horrifying sight. If there is a likelihood of discharge from any of the orifices, they should be packed to protect the family from unpleasant odours or the sight of discharge leaking from the nose or mouth. The hair should be combed carefully, male patients may need shaving, and finger nails should be cleaned and cut.

The shrouding of the body, labelling and preparation for removal to the mortuary vary from hospital to hospital. There is absolutely no reason why requests to dress the body in garments provided by the family should not be granted, but since further cleansing will be performed by the undertaker, relatives may be advised to hand the items of clothing to him.

Many nurses are somewhat aghast when approached by a relative wishing to help with the last offices, finding it morbid and bizarre. Yet it is perfectly natural and understandable that they should want to be involved in this final service to their loved one, and the offer should be welcomed.

REFERENCES

Stedeford, Averil, 'Understanding Confusional States'. *British Journal of Hospital Medicine*, December, 1978.

Breckman, Brigid (ed.), *Stoma Care*. Beaconsfield, 1981.

Chapter 9

Practicalities

The practical advice and information which may be needed by the families and friends of those who are terminally ill is varied and complex. Each patient's financial situation, the existence and ages of his dependants, his housing conditions and the symptoms of his illness will create a unique set of needs. People involved in supporting these families need to regard themselves as a resource which can be drawn upon, if not for specific information and help, then at least for guidance about where it might be obtained.

FINANCIAL AID

One of the greatest sources of anxiety during a prolonged illness, and also after a death, may be shortage of money. Older people, particularly, find it degrading to admit to financial difficulties, and are often reluctant to apply for the assistance to which they are entitled. The health visitor or social worker can help greatly by raising the issue as a matter of course, in a sensitive but business-like manner. Pamphlets about the various types of benefits and allowances can be left for the family to read in privacy. On the next visit, queries may need clearing up and encouragement or help may be necessary to get the application form filled in.

More detailed advice about any of the state pensions can be obtained from the local offices of the Department of Health and Social Security. The whereabouts of these offices and their opening hours should be known to all health care workers. Whilst no one is expected to have detailed knowledge of all the possible benefits, each individual health visitor or district nurse should have her own collection of Department of Health and Social Security pamphlets for reference, and should keep this up to date by paying regular visits to the local Department of Health and Social Security office.

SICKNESS BENEFIT

During an illness, those who have previously been working and have paid national insurance contributions will be eligible for sickness benefit. This is obtained by filling in the back of the medical certificate, now known as the doctor's statement, and sending it to the local Department of Health and Social Security office. This certificate must have been signed by the patient's general practitioner, if the patient is at home, or by authorised hospital personnel, if the patient is in hospital. Sickness benefit is paid for the first twenty-eight weeks of absence from work.

INVALIDITY BENEFIT

At the end of this period, the sickness benefit is replaced by an invalidity benefit, plus an invalidity allowance for women under fifty-five years and men under sixty years. These payments may continue throughout the whole of the patient's potential working life. Additional payments are made for dependants. The change-over from sickness to invalidity benefit is made automatically by the social security officers. Anyone receiving invalidity benefit, although still obliged to submit regular doctor's statements, may be asked by the Department of Health and Social Security to see a Regional Medical Service doctor for examination. However, this is very unlikely in the case of a terminal illness.

OTHER BENEFITS

Additional benefits, to which a family may be entitled when their main bread-winner has a prolonged illness, are supplementary benefit, family income supplement, help with heating costs, free prescriptions, help with hospital fares, and rent and rate rebates. If the family's savings amount to more than the limit allowed, however, these benefits will be prohibited.

ATTENDANCE ALLOWANCE

Attendance allowance is paid to anyone who is no longer capable of caring for himself and who lives at home. After the preliminary application form has been submitted, the patient is assessed at home by a doctor employed by the Department of Health and Social Security.

There are two rates, according to the degree of attention required. The lower rate applies when care is required only during the daytime, whilst the higher rate is given to those needing care both day and night. This allowance is only paid when the patient has satisfied the medical requirements for six months. No back payment is made, and on admission to hospital, the attendance allowance will continue for four weeks only.

MOBILITY ALLOWANCE

The mobility allowance is available to anyone under sixty-five years who is unable (or virtually unable) to walk, and whose doctor considers that he is likely to remain incapacitated for at least a further year. He must, of course, be able to make use of the allowance, i.e. he must be fit enough to be able to travel in a car. This can greatly enrich the life of someone who is terminally ill. The allowance can be used towards hiring or buying a car, when special concessions in hire purchase arrangements and relief from road tax can be obtained. The mobility allowance can be claimed by patients in hospital or institutions, as well as by those living at home.

DEATH GRANT

The death grant is a lump sum of money which is paid to the deceased person's next-of-kin or to the person who is paying for the funeral. The amount varies according to the age of the deceased, less being paid for children and adolescents and those in their late eighties and nineties. Unfortunately, the sum is quite unrealistic in relation to present funeral costs. The death grant can be applied for on the back of the certificate of registration of death. One copy is specially issued for national insurance purposes. If the deceased was married, his marriage certificate should accompany the claim, which must be submitted within six months of death. Even if the funeral is delayed because the body is being used for medical research, the claim should still be made immediately after the death.

Those who find themselves struggling to meet a relative's funeral expenses may be reassured to know that these are one of the first claims on a deceased person's estate.

WIDOW'S ALLOWANCE AND PENSION

Widow's allowance is paid to all widows under sixty years, plus the widows of men who were under sixty-five years when they died, for twenty-six weeks after the death. When this payment ceases, anyone with children under nineteen years, or anyone pregnant at the time of their husband's death, is entitled to a widowed mother's allowance. A widow's pension is paid in full to all widows who are between fifty and sixty years. Those between forty and fifty years receive between thirty and ninety per cent of the pension. This is on a sliding scale, according to age. Common-law wives will receive no widow's benefits at all, however long the couple have been cohabiting. This can seem very unjust at times, especially when the 'wife' has nursed her 'husband' through a long illness. In some cases it may be appropriate for the nurse to point this out before it is too late.

WIDOWER'S BENEFITS

Widowers with children under sixteen years, who decide to give up their employment in order to stay at home and care for their families, are entitled to claim supplementary benefit. This includes a personal allowance, an allowance for each child, which varies according to their age, and a further payment gauged in accordance with the particular family's essential household expenditure. Widowers receive the same benefits as any other one-parent family. If a widowed father decides to take a part-time, lowly-paid job, he is entitled to claim family income supplement. All these benefits are determined by an income and savings assessment, however, and will be withheld if they exceed the limit allowed.

INDUSTRIAL DEATH BENEFIT

Industrial death benefits are paid to the wives and dependants of those who died as a result of an accident at work or from one of the forty or so prescribed industrial diseases. Some forms of cancer come into this category, such as malignant mesothelioma, resulting from asbestosis, and cancer of the bladder and ureter caused by aniline dyes and rubber, and pneumoconiosis from coal dust in the mines.

SICKNESS ABSENTEEISM AND TERMINATION OF EMPLOYMENT

Most employers have a sickness-payment scheme which allows for specific periods of absence through illness, usually six months on full pay, followed by six months on half pay. At the end of this twelve month period, termination of employment is considered. There is no set period of time during which a job must legally be kept open for a person unable to work due to sickness, or for those on compassionate leave whilst caring for a sick relative. The law allows employers to take into account the likelihood of an employee ever becoming fit enough to perform his particular job again and the effect of his absence on his place of work. It would therefore be easier to terminate the employment of someone performing a key role in a small firm, than that of an unskilled worker in a large firm. There are legal requirements, however, about pre-dismissal counselling which generally ensures that patients receive sensitive and careful preparation. Many employers far exceed any legal requirements by providing alternative employment of a less strenuous nature. The ability to continue working in some capacity can do wonders for the morale.

The termination of a dying patient's employment can be a source of great distress. It is such a forceful reminder that there is no hope of recovery and no future. Many firms with a caring approach to staff welfare will treat such cases on individual merit. If they have a policy of considering dismissal after twelve months' absenteeism but the employee concerned is already critically ill by that time, no action will be taken and payment of half his salary often continues.

OTHER SOURCES OF INCOME

Although the number and variety of benefits seem vast, the amount of money paid to any one family or individual is far from excessive. Savings are soon swallowed up and those who have none may be hard-pressed to make ends meet. For this reason, it may be necessary to direct people towards other possible sources of income from charitable organisations. The local Council of Voluntary Services can often provide information about local charitable bodies who might be able to offer financial aid.

Cancer patients in financial need are eligible for help from the National Society for Cancer Relief (a national charity) with any extra costs incurred as a result of the disease. The Society does not deal direct with patients, as so many are not aware of the nature of their illness. Applications to the Society should be made by a social worker, health visitor or community nurse. Any reasonable request is considered if it is for the benefit of the patient or his immediate family during the patient's lifetime. However, all grants are subject to a strict assessment of income and savings, so that help is directed only to those people with low incomes. Anyone working with cancer patients should carry a supply of application forms. These can be obtained from the Benefits Department of the National Society for Cancer Relief. Some of the self-help groups, such as the Leukaemia Society and the National Association of Laryngectomee Clubs will also give financial help to those in need. (Addresses are given on page 201.)

The social services department is the best source of help and advice in cases of financial hardship, having discretionary powers to give immediate financial assistance to those in urgent need.

WHO HELPS AT HOME?

However highly motivated a family may be to care for their dying relative at home, without the right kind of help it may well prove impossible. The quality and quantity of services available varies enormously from area to area. Fortunately, in the rural areas, where services tend to be minimal, the involvement of the local community is usually far more evident, though not always.

The development of specialist home care services was described on page 9 since it is a major component of the hospice movement, but their role should not be forgotten when considering those who help at home.

THE GENERAL PRACTITIONER

The general practitioner has a vital role to play in managing a terminal illness, not only in the detailed attention to symptom control, but also in communication regarding the diagnosis, prognosis and treatment, and in the provision of emotional support for both the patient and family. He will be responsible for enlisting the help of the community nurses and health visitor when he feels this to be appropriate. In no other way is the doctor's concern, involvement and support expressed as effectively as in a home visit, however time consuming this may be. Unfortunately, some general practitioners are so discomforted by feelings of embarrassment, inadequacy and failure when with their dying patients that home visits may be either avoided altogether, or else they are short and superficial, often consisting of the briefest of greetings. Of course most general practitioners are extremely busy and it is often the size of their workload, as much as their lack of motivation, which prevents them from visiting as often as they should.

The health visitor or community nurse can sometimes encourage home calls by constantly initiating discussion about the patient, reporting back any changes in his symptoms or mental state, and by telling the general practitioner how much the family value his visits. Nurses have a responsibility to support and encourage their colleagues as well as their patients, and this includes the doctor, who is too often excluded because he is considered to be self-sufficient.

THE HEALTH VISITOR

The health visitor has a very broad role. She may well have known the family for many years, particularly if there are young children. She, too, will provide counselling and emotional support, which will continue during the time of bereavement. She will be responsible for liaising with all the other services, as and when their particular help is needed. She can advise on financial matters and organise the provision of any equipment which is needed. The health visitor will help tackle all manner of individual family problems. If there are young children, she will discuss how best to explain to them what is happening and how best to support them. This may involve a visit to the school to make sure that their teacher is fully aware of the situation and is making the necessary allowances. If there is an elderly relative being cared for, as well as the person who is dying, she may be able to arrange a holiday admission to 'Part 3' accommodation.

In some areas, the health visitor's role is still confined to families with young children. This is changing, however, especially where primary care teams are all based together in health centres. Where it is not happening, health visitors should be reminding their medical colleagues of their wider role.

COMMUNITY NURSES

The community nurses, still known by most people as district nurses, will visit when physical nursing care is required. This may be to perform dressings, bowel management, catheter care, injections or all manner of other specific treatments. If the patient becomes too weak to care for himself, they will perform basic nursing care each day. During the last few weeks of life, they are often visiting three times a day to turn the patient, give mouth care, and administer pain-relieving suppositories or injections. Some areas provide a night nursing service, but even where these are in existence they are usually fairly minimal.

NIGHT NURSES/SITTERS

Night sitters are occasionally organised by local voluntary groups, though they may receive some payment from the National Society for Cancer Relief or other charities. For the relative who has been caring for someone both day and night for many weeks, the value of one or two nights of unbroken sleep, when they are not having to listen out for their sick relative, is enormous. In fact, this is frequently the factor which makes or breaks the possibility of home care. Unfortunately, these night sitters are few and far between. The establishment of night sitting services would seem to be an important extension of the work of local hospices, and one which should be given high priority when future development is planned. Marie Curie nurses are available to care for terminally ill patients at night in some areas, and even where they do not exist, the Trust will often pay the salary of a local nurse if one can be obtained. (Address given on page 201.) This is usually organised through the 'nurse bank' of the district health authority.

SOCIAL WORKERS

A social worker will not necessarily be involved with all dying patients, unless there are problems which require her particular expertise. These may be practical matters of finance, housing, or the care of dependants, but will just as frequently be emotional difficulties, regarding relationships or adjustment to the expectation of a short prognosis, for example. Her role may overlap with that of the health visitor, and in some cases she will perform many of the tasks previously ascribed to the health visitor. Where young families are concerned, the need for both practical help and emotional support is so great that both disciplines can be usefully employed, and ideally they would provide support for one another.

The social worker can be contacted by the general practitioner, the health visitor or the district nurse, but any patient or relative can telephone or visit the social services department themselves to ask for help.

DOMICILIARY OCCUPATIONAL THERAPIST

The domiciliary occupational therapist plays a vital role in helping to maintain the patient's independence for as long as possible. Much of her work will be concerned with assessing the patient's needs, the provision of equipment and aids, and master-minding alterations in the home. As such, it is described more fully in the section 'Equipment, Aids and Adaptations' on page 195.

Domiciliary occupational therapists may be based in health centres or in departments of community medicine or nursing. Patients are referred to them by general practitioners, social workers, health visitors or community nurses.

DOMICILIARY PHYSIOTHERAPIST

The domiciliary physiotherapists could make a valuable contribution to the care of the terminally ill, but their scarcity prevents this in most areas. Where they are available, their help is sought most frequently in mobilising patients who are no longer able to walk without aids, who have suffered a pathological fracture, or who have had a long period in bed. Patients with paralysis also benefit greatly from the attention of a physiotherapist, as she can help to relieve painful muscle spasms and contractures by putting their limbs through a full range of passive movements. The general practitioner, district nurse or health visitor are responsible for referring patients to the domiciliary physiotherapist.

SPEECH THERAPIST

A few terminally ill patients will have severe speech problems. The main groups will be those who have had cerebrovascular accidents and those suffering from one of the degenerative diseases, particularly motor neurone disease. Speech therapists, although valuable, are again very thin on the ground, and treatment can often be given only to those patients who are fit enough to travel to the speech therapy department of the local hospital. Patients are referred for speech therapy by their general practitioner.

HOME HELPS

Home helps can relieve the caring relative of many of his household chores, so that he has more time and energy to devote to the patient. They will also provide tremendous companionship and emotional support. In the case of a dying patient living alone, the home help is often the most important person involved in their care, frequently undertaking tasks far in excess of those for which she is paid. The home help organiser is always based in the local social services department. Some payment, determined by an income assessment, may be required from the family.

Referrals can be made by any member of the primary care team, by a social worker or by the patient himself.

MINISTERS OF RELIGION

The help given by the minister of religion does not normally come into the category of practical help, since his main role is the provision of spiritual and emotional support. In some parishes, however, it may well be the local minister who first perceives what a family's needs are and mobilises the church community to meet them. He is very likely to know the best people to approach for the different types of help which may be needed, and can provide an invaluable link with the community for the caring professionals who are unfamiliar with the locality.

VOLUNTEERS

Many voluntary organisations offer a great deal of help to the families of very ill patients. These vary from area to area, but the Citizen's Advice Bureau or Council of Voluntary Services will be able to give detailed, local information. Most areas have church groups or 'Good Neighbour' and 'Fish' schemes. These provide volunteers to sit with patients, enabling their relatives to have a few hours off to go shopping or to visit the hairdresser, for instance. They may also provide transport for hospital appointments or hospital visiting, or just to take the sick person out for a drive. They will usually collect prescriptions or other shopping, and if the sick person lives alone, will often prepare hot drinks and meals and even help with household chores such as laying fires and gardening. The Women's Royal Voluntary Service and the Red Cross are better known for their work in hospitals, in running clothing stores for those in hardship, and in fund-raising. However, they also provide volunteers in many areas to sit with or help care for sick people at home. The Red Cross makes two other valuable contributions by running courses in home nursing for the general public, and providing stores of nursing apparatus for loan to anyone being nursed at home. (Addresses are given on page 202.)

MEALS ON WHEELS

In most areas, a meals on wheels service provides a hot meal on every weekday or on alternate weekdays. Premises and food are usually provided by the local authority, whilst voluntary organisations do the cooking and delivering, but this varies from area to area. The quality of the meals, although often very good, is sometimes spoiled by the length of time between being prepared and being eaten. They are consequently under constant criticism by many of the elderly people who receive them. However, for the elderly patient living alone, this may be their main source of nourishment. Needless to say, a piece of steamed fish, a bowl of home-made soup or an egg custard is often far more palatable and suitable for someone who is terminally ill. Neighbours are sometimes willing to help in this way, although they may need encouragement from the community nurse or health visitor, as people are frequently afraid of offending the sick person's pride.

LAUNDRY SERVICE

If patients are incontinent, the free laundry service can be invaluable. This involves the provision of a constant supply of clean bed-linen and the removal of soiled laundry. This linen is loaned by the social services department of the local authority, which funds the laundry; none of the patient's own bedding or clothing is removed. However, this service is only available in a limited number of urban areas. Washing six sheets a day, plus clothes and other bedding, can be the last straw for many relatives. It is not only exhausting, but also expensive and time-consuming. The use of waterproof undersheets, incontinence pads and pants can help to reduce the laundry problem considerably. If soiled incontinence sheets, dressing pads or colostomy bags cannot be burned, bags marked 'for incineration' are supplied by the local health authority. These are taken away and incinerated by the normal local authority refuse collectors.

AFTER-CARE

Although the primary care team, the medical social worker and the minister of religion will continue to visit and offer their support to the family after the patient has died, many of the other agencies of help will no longer be appropriate. There are some voluntary organisations which provide help specifically for the bereaved. 'Cruse' is one such organisation with branches all over the country. In addition to the social gatherings, where great comfort can be gained from meeting others in the same situation, talks are arranged on many useful topics, such as home electricity, car maintenance, cooking for one, and legal matters. All branches also provide a counselling service, with an interview appointment system, twenty-four-hour telephone counsellors, and in some areas, home visits on request.

The Gingerbread organisation runs along similar lines, but is specifically for one-parent families. These may be the result of death, but are more often the result of separation or divorce. Both of these groups are frequently thought to be available to widows only but are, in fact, equally available and just as valuable to widowers. The Society of Compassionate Friends is another self-help organisation run by and for the parents of children with a fatal disease and those whose children have died.

The Samaritans are now well-known, providing a telephone service throughout Britain for those in despair, particularly for anyone who is contemplating suicide. Many of their calls are from the newly-bereaved, some of whom also use the Samaritans face-to-face counselling service. (The addresses of these and other organisations which help the bereaved are given on page 202.)

EQUIPMENT, AIDS AND ADAPTATIONS

In order to keep a patient in as much comfort as possible, to help him to maintain the maximum degree of independence, and to minimise the physical strain of nursing on his family, a wide variety of medical aids will be needed. The health visitor and community nurse will have detailed knowledge of what is available and will be able to match this information to their assessment of the patient's needs. If a more expert assessment is considered to be necessary, the domiciliary occupational therapist will visit and advise. Most equipment can be obtained on loan from either the community section of the health authority or the local branch of the Red Cross.

The following are those items most commonly required, but many other more specific aids are available to help with particular disabilities:
a) hospital beds, back rests, bed boards, foot boards, bed cradles, bed tables, bed elevators, hoists, screens;
b) high-backed chairs, reclining chairs, wheel chairs (self-propelling or electric), foot stools;

c) ripple beds and cushions, air-rings, sheepskin sheets, bootees and elbow muffs;

d) walking frames, tripods, crutches, walking sticks;

e) bath seats, non-slip bath mats, raised lavatory seats, lavatory frames with arms, commodes, bedpans, urinals, waterproof undersheets, incontinence pants and pads;

f) adapted feeding utensils, hand bells, long-handled shoe horns, pick-up-sticks;

g) electric fans (including those with deodorising action), portable radios and televisions (the latter with remote control), compression pumps for swollen limbs, intercom systems, liquidisers. (Some of the items in this group are not available for loan from the health authority or Red Cross, but Social Services can sometimes obtain them.)

If any of these items are required, they are usually needed fairly urgently; unfortunately, there is frequently a delay in obtaining some of them. With patients who are terminally ill, this may well mean that they arrive too late to be of any use. Some of the money donated to the hospices could be profitably used to fund a pool of equipment reserved exclusively for loan to the terminally ill.

Many patients find difficulty in dressing themselves unless their clothes are adapted a little. The hospital or domiciliary occupational therapist will usually advise, and even get alterations done in the Occupational Therapy department if there is no one else to help. Buttons and hooks and eyes can usually be replaced quite easily by Velcro, and most waist-bands can be elasticated. Loose kaftan-style dresses, smock tops, wrap-around skirts and capes are very worthwhile investments for female patients. Men can prove more difficult to help unless they are willing to abandon their collar and tie in favour of open-neck shirts and polo-neck sweaters.

If minor adaptations to the home are necessary, such as ramps for wheelchairs or handrails for the bath or lavatory, the domiciliary occupational therapist will make a home visit to assess the need, and will then arrange for the work to be done. If more major work is necessary, such as the building of a downstairs bathroom when a patient is no longer able to get upstairs, the social worker will need to be involved. She will be able to advise on applying for grants, and in the case of council houses, will liaise with the housing department about getting the work done. It would be irresponsible to put pressure on the authorities to get major, structural work done for someone known to have a very short prognosis but, occasionally, people who are terminally ill will warrant such action.

WILLS

Making a will when someone is terminally ill can be a most painful process. For this reason, it is always beneficial to have made one well in advance when it does not hold such ominous implications. It is, of course, important to make it correctly so that it can actually be implemented. If the making of the will is left until the person concerned is critically ill, and a solicitor is used, the cost of home or hospital visits can be very high indeed. Although it is quite possible to draw up a will without the assistance of a solicitor, unless one is extremely well-informed on the subject it is far safer to pay the quite reasonable fee for legal advice. Solicitors make more profit from sorting out wills which have been incorrectly made than from drawing them up initially. Having made an appointment with a solicitor, it is a good idea to list all one's assets, taking along any relevant documents such as life insurance policies or mortgage agreements. Another list needs to be drawn up of those people who are to benefit from the will, with the item or amount of money they are to receive. The names and addresses of one or two people willing to act as executors will also be required. These can be anyone over the age of eighteen years. Many people name their next-of-kin as one, and their bank or solicitor as the other. The executors are responsible for sorting out and distributing the estate after a death and they can be beneficiaries. Two witnesses have to sign the will, but neither of these may be beneficiaries.

Once the will is completed, it is usual to leave one copy with the solicitor or in the bank, keeping the other in a safe place in the home. The executor should be informed of the whereabouts of at least one copy.

Immediately after a death has occurred, the executors must take the will to the Probate Office. Once it has been checked for legality and officially authorised by the Probate Registrar, the executors are entitled to execute it. If neither executor has any legal knowledge, it is once again advisable to seek the help of a solicitor, particularly where property is involved. It is in the execution of a will that heavy legal fees may be incurred, but the absence of advice can lead to far worse problems. It is essential to review a will every five years or so, in case the estate or the situation has changed drastically. One example is the event of a marriage, when any previous will is revoked.

WHAT TO DO AFTER A DEATH

If someone dies at home, the family doctor will normally give the relative or next-of-kin the death certificate at the time he comes to certify the death. If someone dies in hospital, the relative will probably be asked to come to the hospital the following morning to collect the patient's personal property and the medical certificate of death. The hospital staff or family doctor will need to know whether the patient is to be buried or cremated, because a separate certificate, signed by two doctors, is required for cremation. This is given to the undertaker.

A post mortem may be requested if the death was unexpected, if the primary cause of the disease was never found, if the case was unusual in any way or if the patient was admitted to hospital less than twenty-four hours before the death occurred. If the request is made by the patient's doctor the next-of-kin may refuse, but if the coroner requests a post mortem, with or without an inquest, the next-of-kin has no legal right to refuse permission. This may delay the funeral for several days, which can be very disturbing for the family. Many people are horrified by the thought of the body of their loved one being cut open, and need a great deal of additional support to cope with it. They are often very reassured to hear that all incisions are sutured once the post mortem has been completed.

If death occurs in hospital, the family and friends may view the body in the mortuary chapel, if they wish to. The fact that the body has just been removed from a refrigerator and is, therefore, extremely cold, can be very upsetting to anyone who has not been prepared. It is important for a member of the nursing staff to check the appearance of the body before the family see it. So often the sight of dishevelled hair or discharge from the mouth or nose can leave the relatives with distressing memories. It is often kindest to suggest that relatives wait to view the body until it is in the undertaker's chapel of rest, where the environment is usually far more comforting than the hospital mortuary.

The death should be registered within five days of its occurrence by the Registrar of Births and Deaths of the area in which it occurred. The medical certificate of death should be taken, plus the deceased person's medical card. The latter is simply to update the National Health Service register. If it cannot be found immediately, an addressed envelope is supplied by the Registrar to post it on later. There is no need to make an appointment to register the death in most areas, as the next-of-kin or his representative can simply go along during opening hours.

Copies of the death certificate can be obtained as soon as the registration is completed. It is a good idea to record the number of the entry in the register and the date, in case further copies have to be applied for later.

If it is appropriate, the minister of religion should be contacted next, if he was not present at the death. In most cases he will visit the family at home the same day, and as well as offering spiritual comfort, will begin to make arrangements for the funeral. Most ministers are only too pleased to include any favourite hymns, prayers, readings or references to particular attributes of the deceased, which the family suggest.

At this point the undertaker should also be approached. An appointment can be made, either to go to the undertaker's office, or for him to visit the home. The cost of a funeral varies greatly, but it can be very high indeed. For this reason it is often useful for someone who is not so distressed by the death, such as a friend or relative, to be present at the interview. A price list should always be seen.

Any requests about garments of clothing for the deceased to be dressed in, the removal or replacement of rings, and whether or not the body is to be embalmed, should be raised. Embalming involves the replacement of blood with formalin in order to delay the process of decomposition. This makes the handling of the body far less distasteful for the undertaker and is, therefore, often carried out (and charged for) without any prior discussion with the family. If this service is not required, it should be stated at the initial interview.

It is usual for the undertaker to collect the body from the home or hospital, to cleanse and embalm it, and to construct a coffin of the material chosen by the family. Arrangements will be made with either the cemetery or the crematorium, and the fees paid in advance. The undertaker will also pay the minister of religion, the organist, the choir master and the grave diggers. A hearse and pall bearers will take the body to the church or the cemetery or crematorium. In the event of a cremation, he will also be responsible for disposing of the ashes. This may be by burial in a casket, or the family may wish to scatter them themselves. The choice of a plaque or sculpture for the grave will have an enormous effect on the overall cost of the funeral. Most undertakers will also make arrangements for newspaper announcements, funeral cars, floral tributes and catering for a meal after the service, but these items may be far less expensive if organised independently by the family. Viewing the body at the undertaker's is quite usual, but an appointment system is generally in use. The body will be displayed inside the coffin, dressed in a white shroud.

Many people choose to leave their bodies to medical research departments or schools of anatomy. This can be arranged by the person concerned long before his death, by contacting the professor of anatomy at the nearest university or medical school. The latter should be informed immediately after the death has occurred. If they accept the body, they will arrange for its removal once the necessary forms have been completed. If the death occurs at a great distance from the research or teaching centre, the latter may refuse to accept the body because of the cost of transport. If the corneas of the eyes or any other organs are donated, they will need to be removed immediately. The body is then returned to the family for burial or cremation. In the former instance, when the whole body is donated, the remains will be returned for burial only if specifically requested. More bodies are bequeathed than are needed at present. For this reason, the bodies of many donors who die of malignant disease are not accepted, as the anatomy is often grossly distorted.

One reason frequently given for donating a body is to escape the necessity of a religious service, when neither the deceased nor his family had a specific faith. This is not necessary, however, as the body can be buried or cremated without any service at all, although the permission of the incumbent of the parish is required in the case of burial in a churchyard. Alternatively, a non-religious ceremony, possibly containing an address about the deceased, with music, poetry readings and silent contemplation, can be organised by the family and friends.

REFERENCES

What To Do When Someone Dies. The Consumer's Association, 1978.
The Charities Digest, 1982. The Family Welfare Association.
Social Security leaflets, issued by the DHSS, 1982.
The Disabilities Rights Handbook, 1982, issued by the DHSS.

USEFUL ADDRESSES

FINANCIAL HELP

The National Society for Cancer Relief. Michael Sobell House, 30 Dorset Square, London NW1 6QL. Tel. 01-402 8125

NURSING AND MEDICAL CARE AT HOME AND IN HOSPICES

The National Society for Cancer Relief. (Address and telephone number as above)

Marie Curie Memorial Foundation. 124 Sloane Street, London SW1 9BP. Tel. 01-730 9157

The Sue Ryder Foundation. Cavendish, Suffolk, CO10 8AY. Tel. 0787-280252

PRACTICAL HELP

The Disabled Living Foundation (provides an advisory service on the aids available for the disabled). 346 Kensington High Street, London W14. Tel. 01-602 2491

PATIENTS' SELF-HELP GROUPS

(offering information, social events, counselling and, in some cases, financial assistance)

Colostomy Welfare Group. 38-39 Eccleston Square, 2nd Floor, London SW1V 1PB. Tel. 01-828 5175

The National Association of Laryngectomee Clubs. Fourth Floor, Michael Sobell House, 30 Dorset Square, London NW1 6QL. Tel. 01-402 6007

Leukaemia Society. 45 Craigmoor Avenue, Queen's Park, Bournemouth, Dorset. Tel. 0202-37459

Multiple Sclerosis Society of Great Britain and Northern Ireland. 4 Tachbrook Street, London SW1V 1SJ. Tel. 01-834 8231/2/3

Motor Neurone Disease Association. 17 Lorimer Avenue, Gedling, Nottingham NG4 4BS. Tel. 0602-878700

Mastectomy Association. 25 Brighton Road, South Croydon, Surrey CR2 6EA. Tel. 01-654 8643

CARE. (Cancer Aftercare and Rehabilitation Education) Lodge Cottage, Church Lane, Tinsbury, Bath, Somerset. Tel. 0761-70731

ORGANISATIONS FOR THE BEREAVED

Cruse (there are local branches in most areas) 126 Sheen Road, Richmond, Surrey TW9 1CR. Tel. 01-940 4818/9047

The Society of Compassionate Friends. 50 Woodwaye, Watford, Hertfordshire. Tel. 0923-24279

Gingerbread. 35 Wellington Street, London WC2. Tel. 01-240 0953

The National Association of Widows. Stafford District Voluntary Service Centre, Chell Road, Stafford ST16 2QA. Tel. 0785-45465

The National Council for the Single Woman and Her Dependants. NCSWD Ltd., 29 Chilworth Mews, London W2 3RG. Tel. 01-262 1451/2

British Guild for Sudden Infant Death Study. Pathology Department, Royal Infirmary, Cardiff CF2 1SZ. Tel. 0222-492233

OTHER RELEVANT ORGANISATIONS

British Red Cross. 9 Grosvenor Crescent, London SW1X 7EJ. Tel. 01-235 5454

WRVS (Women's Royal Voluntary Service) 17 Old Park Lane, London W1Y 4AJ. Tel. 01-499 6040

The Samaritans. 17 Uxbridge Road, Slough SL1 1SN. Tel. 0753-32713/4

'Hospice Information'. St Christopher's Hospice, 51-53 Lawrie Park Road, Sydenham, London SE26 6DZ. Tel. 01-778 1240

Chapter 10

Euthanasia and Suicide

Voluntary euthanasia is described as the painless ending of life at the request of the person concerned, when suffering is intolerable and cannot be relieved. It is a sad reflection on Western society that euthanasia is the first thought which springs to the mind of many people when the care of the dying is mentioned. This is, no doubt, tied up with our culture of death denial.

The Voluntary Euthanasia Society, now renamed EXIT, has become an increasingly large and powerful pressure group since its foundation in 1935, the main aim of the society being the provision of legislation for voluntary euthanasia. To date, no such legislation has been passed either in Britain or in any other country, but the Suicide Act of 1961 has made it seem more likely that it may exist one day. Although the prime concern of this Act was to prevent suicide from continuing to be a criminal offence, thereby showing compassion for those who had 'failed', in so doing it inevitably gave expression to a legal disregard for the sanctity of life.

EXIT is presently concentrating on ways of assisting people to commit suicide as painlessly and effectively as possible, with the least distress to the individual as well as to the survivors. The booklet which they have prepared, outlining some of the methods of doing so, has caused great controversy, not least because of the danger of such information being made available to potential murderers and the emotionally unstable.

As the law now stands, administering a drug or following any other procedure, deliberately and specifically to accelerate death, even to end the suffering of an incurable patient, is classified as murder; that is, the unlawful killing of a human being with malice aforethought, expressed, or implied. Since the law holds that the intention to kill is always malicious, such 'compassionate' action cannot even be categorised as manslaughter, since this term only applies to an unpremeditated killing.

EUTHANASIA AND THE TERMINALLY ILL

Those with slowly progressive degenerative diseases, severe senile dementia, or any other condition where mental or physical function is irreparably impaired, may have a strong case in support of voluntary euthanasia, but their position is very different from those with a terminal illness and a relatively short prognosis. However, a number of the terminally ill also think about the possibility of euthanasia for a variety of reasons. Amongst these are intractable pain, immobility, disfigurement, incontinence or any of the other harrowing aspects of disease. For some, their mental anguish, such as the fear of dying, the grief of anticipated loss, or confusion, makes life seem intolerable. Mental anguish also embraces the pain of dependency, the feeling of worthlessness, and the knowledge that one is becoming a physical and financial burden on one's family. Any combination of these factors can produce a quality of life which some people find unacceptable. The widely held belief that the eventual death from disease will be more painful than euthanasia may well be the final trigger. Many of these reasons can be eliminated by skilled care, and death occurring naturally can almost always be as painless as euthanasia, so long as drugs are used in the appropriate manner.

Nevertheless, some severe physical and mental suffering cannot be relieved, so do we have the right to insist on the continuation of such a life? Large quantities of money, at present spent on the care of the dying, could be redirected to improve the quality of life for the living. Should the religious beliefs of a minority about the sanctity of human life be imposed upon the whole of society? Does a man's life belong to himself, to the society in which he lives, or to his God? Does personal liberty justify the right to decide whether or not to have one's life curtailed? There are no finite answers to these questions.

The instinct for survival is so powerful that, even if legalised, euthanasia would undoubtedly be rejected by many of those who now request it. When given the very best care possible, the majority of dying patients are longing for a few months more, not less. There is no doubt that the availability of euthanasia would create an enormous torment for the dying, many of whom are only too aware of the work, the cost, and the mental suffering that their condition is causing.

No doctor is called upon to prolong the dying of a patient with a fatal illness. Much of the pressure for euthanasia has undoubtedly been encouraged by the failure of the medical profession to acknowledge when enough curative treatment is enough. Doctors are authorised to give drugs in the doses required to relieve pain and distress. In some cases there is no doubt that this necessitates rendering the patient unconscious, which in turn frequently leads to pulmonary congestion and subsequent pneumonia. The death which ensues is not classified as euthanasia, as the drug was given with the honest intention of relieving pain, and the acceleration of death was just an unavoidable side-effect. This practice seems acceptable to most people and has been openly condoned by the Vatican.

SUICIDE

Many courageous patients with terminal disease take their own lives each year. This is usually achieved by overdosage with drugs which are frequently prescribed in excessive quantities (enough for several weeks at a time, rather than high doses) and with inadequate supervision. It is possible that a great many more people die in this way than is ever discovered or disclosed, since their deaths could so easily be accounted for by the fatal disease from which they were suffering.

However, many suicides are performed in a messy and degrading manner, leaving grotesque memories in the minds of those who discover them. Some attempts, although equally undignified, are unsuccessful. Both of these possibilities are usually the result of inadequate information or materials, since painless and dignified ways of ending one's own life do exist. A large percentage of suicide attempts are cries for help, but those occurring amongst the terminally ill are generally the result of a firm determination to curtail the dying process. So are we right to prevent EXIT from making this vital information available? Doctors, with full insight into their own medical condition, detailed knowledge of how they might end their lives in a dignified manner, and free access to the necessary drugs, have the highest suicide rate of any occupational group.

One section of the community for whom suicide is not an option is comprised of those whose physical disability renders them incapable even of taking pills unaided. Should euthanasia be made available to people with this degree of handicap? If it were, what would we be telling them about the value society places upon their lives? How many would feel obliged to accept it, conscious of the burden they are imposing on their families, regardless of their own wishes?

There are many patients who would never consciously consider suicide, but who succeed in shortening their lives by refusing treatment or food (see also page 168). Although including in this section of the book, refusing to eat or drink or refusing to accept treatment, and thereby allowing nature to take its course, is not usually considered to be suicide.

Even during the earlier stages of a fatal illness, some patients will exercise their right to refuse treatment. The medical staff may believe that there is still some hope of cure, or at least of palliating the disease. Nevertheless, if the patient feels that his quality of life is such that any prolongation would be undesirable, he cannot be treated against his will. Most doctors in this situation would try very hard to persuade the patient to change his mind but, if that were not possible, they would respect his wishes. Although no doctor would find this easy to accept, their commitment to the patient will usually be strong enough to ensure that they remain closely involved, continuing to provide symptom control where necessary.

Occasionally, nursing staff may feel that patients are being bludgeoned into accepting treatment that they really do not want. If the doctors and nurses concerned trust and respect one another, differences of opinion will usually be heeded. If this is not the case, and patients' rights are apparently being undermined, it is essential that the matter is reported to a more senior level of authority.

WHO REQUESTS EUTHANASIA?

Contrary to popular belief, requests for euthanasia by those with a terminal illness are not common. As stated earlier, the most frequently expressed desire is for more time, not less. Nurses are far more likely to encounter this problem when nursing the elderly or the chronic sick. By contrasting a typical situation of someone with a chronic disease with that of a person who is terminally ill, the reason for this discrepancy becomes clearer.

Take, for example, a woman in her mid-sixties who has already had fifteen years of pain and increasing disability caused by rheumatoid arthritis. She is now widowed and has no children and no close friends or relatives. She knows that she may live for another twenty years or more, but what has she to look forward to? Every movement produces excruciating pain, and she cannot remember when she last slept for more than two hours without being woken by pain. She is already in a wheelchair, needs help with washing, dressing and toiletting and she cannot write or sew. She will soon have to give up her home and move into an institution. She has always been a very active, practical person, with little interest in music or reading. She has also been a very private, independent person and the thought of being dependent on other people to this extent is intolerable. It is hardly surprising that she contemplates ways of ending her life.

Now let us look at a man in his late fifties with a rapidly growing carcinoma of the bronchus. He has a wife, one daughter and three grandchildren. His main symptoms are anorexia, weakness and a cough which produces a moderate degree of chest pain. Unlike the previous patient, his symptoms can all be relieved to a great extent. (This is partly to do with the length of his prognosis. The side-effects of steroids and narcotics, for example, need not concern those who are prescribing them for short periods.) Knowing that he is likely to die within a few months and feeling reasonably well, there seems a great deal to do. There are people and places he wants to see for what may be the last time. He wants to enjoy his grandchildren's company. He wants to sort through all his personal effects, clearing out a life-time's collection of clutter. He wants to put his business affairs in order, making sure that his wife understands everything to do with their home and financial position. He may want to distribute some of his possessions or revise his will. He may decide to take a world cruise with his wife, or visit his brother in New Zealand. It is hardly surprising that his plea is for a few months more rather than less.

Of course these examples are both extreme cases, to emphasize the point that is being made. Many of the chronically sick are capable of living rich and contented lives, whilst many of the terminally ill cannot face life with a death sentence hanging over them. Nevertheless, they are both true cases and neither is particularly unusual. This would indicate that the hospice movement, with its aim of improving the care of the dying, does not offer an alternative to those most likely to request euthanasia.

THE NURSE'S RESPONSE

Dying patients do sometimes express a longing for death, even when they are receiving the best care possible, but requests for euthanasia are far more likely to come from relatives. This happens most frequently at the very end of life, often after the patient has lost consciousness. The stertorous respirations and other unfamiliar sounds which emanate from the deeply unconscious can, understandably, be interpreted as expressions of great suffering. Relatives frequently ask nurses to put the dying person out of his misery, almost invariably adding, 'No animal would ever be allowed to suffer in this way'.

The nurse can only respond by reassuring the relatives that the symptoms they find so distressing are not indications of pain. This will be far more convincing if regular analgesics are still being given, either by injection or in suppository form. The relative's request, however, may simply be his way of saying that he cannot take any more. The following piece of dialogue took place under just these conditions. Sam was the patient's son. He was about thirty years old and worked in the hospital as a laboratory technician. He had just been very angry and abusive towards a junior nurse, following the most trivial incident of clumsiness on her part.

Sister: Do you think it might help to tell me what's making you so angry?

Sam: I'm sorry. Yes, I would like to ask you something.

Sister: Shall we go down to my office for a bit of privacy?

Sam: I don't really know how to put it . . . it sounds so ungrateful after all the wonderful care you're giving Dad and all the kindness everyone has shown to Mum and us lot. In fact I don't think I can ask you at all. It's so unfair to put you in such a position.

Sister: Well, at least try me. You've no idea how tedious non-stop gratitude can get.

Sam: Well, it's just . . . well I know Dad's got cancer of the kidney and that it's spread to his liver and, well, that his whole condition is incurable, irreversible, in fact he's just dying. That's true isn't it?

Sister: I'm afraid so.

Sam: I don't know a great deal about medicine, in fact I don't know anything at all, but I gather that if Dad were on just about any other type of ward, they would have set up drips and tubes to feed him and keep him hydrated, probably keeping him alive for several more weeks. Am I right?

Sister: Yes, that's absolutely true. But as we all tend to see things here, when disease is as extensive, painful and debilitating as it is in your father's case, that kind of action is quite inappropriate. In fact, it would be prolonging dying, not life.

Sam: I'm with you all the way. I'm not criticising on that score at all. So here you allow nature to take its course. But you also give drugs, don't you?

Sister: Yes we do, for pain or any other symptoms.

Sam: What I'm trying to get at is – why does Dad have to go through these last days at all? He's just getting more deeply unconscious, just like an animal. Why do Mum and my brothers and I have to spend these agonising days and hours just watching him degenerate before our eyes? He looks so bloody awful. Why do you give him just a certain level of sedation, but not enough to bring a merciful end for all of us? Oh God, you must think I'm evil wishing my own father dead, just because I can't cope any longer. What a terrible thing to say when you've done everything in your power to make it bearable for us. I must be going mad. I just don't know what I'm saying any more.

Sister: I'm quite sure you're not going mad. I've heard these same questions too often before to think that. There's nothing evil about it either. If you didn't care about your father, I'm quite sure you wouldn't be asking these questions.

Sam: How much longer can it go on for?

Sister: I don't think it will be many more hours.

Sam: Why can't you just put an end to it now?

Sister: This isn't any consolation, but I can only give what the doctors prescribe and they are forbidden by law to give drugs for the purpose of ending life. They can only give an adequate dose to relieve pain and distress or, if this proves impossible, to render unconscious, as we have in your father's case.

Sam: Where's the moral in that? God, who dreams up laws like that? It should be people like you, who really know what it's all about, making those kind of laws. What virtue is there in making someone unconscious but keeping them alive? It's crazy.

Sister: I know that this time is quite unbearable for you, because it seems so meaningless and useless. I've found myself asking the same questions very often. But for your mother these few days have been valuable. She has worked through so much – through her original denial of what was happening, through anger and bitterness, and is now so composed and prepared for his death.

Sam: You're right. She's suddenly become so strong. I never thought she'd cope so well. That makes me even more ashamed of this outburst. You know I haven't been able to face going into Dad's room all day today, yet she hasn't left his side for more than five minutes.

Sister: Would you like me to come in with you now?

Sam: If you would. Have you ever had to deal with such a hopeless coward before?

Sister: Yes, every day – me.

When patients themselves ask about euthanasia, it is sometimes to clarify in their own minds what kind of response they will receive. Many people are unsure of the present legal position, and some will have heard accounts of illegal practice taking place. Consequently, there are patients who will be relieved to discover that euthanasia is not an option.

It is up to the nurse concerned to discover exactly why a patient is asking about euthanasia. Almost invariably it transpires that they have no wish to end their lives at present, but that fears of unrelieved pain and suffering to come make them anxious to know that euthanasia will be there as a possible escape route. An honest description of what dying is really like, and information about the way in which any likely symptoms will be controlled, can sometimes reduce the fears considerably.

Unfortunately, there are still some patients whose mental or physical suffering cannot be relieved. Some doctors do not have the necessary expertise in using the wide range of drugs available, whilst others are too concerned about addiction or side-effects to prescribe adequate doses, and some pain is simply not amenable to any of the available treatments. This was the case in the following account.

A doctor of medicine in his early sixties was dying from carcinoma of the oesophagus. He had a tracheostomy tube in situ, but the tumour was growing fast and he had nearly died three times from respiratory obstruction. Each time he had been resuscitated and the tube reinserted. During the second of these respiratory arrests, anoxia had caused permanent brain damage which resulted in expressive aphasia.

The doctor's wife had a long history of depressive illness. Although she had coped remarkably well with her husband's illness to date, the appearance of the tumour, which was now fungating around his throat, his inability to communicate with her, and his fear, which was becoming so apparent, were proving to be more than she could tolerate.

His fear of suffocation was overwhelming. This was hardly surprising when one considered that he had been through it three times already. He told the doctors, in written notes, that he could not face another day in this condition, and asked them to sedate him. His anxiety was so great that despite frequent adjustments in the dose, and variations in the type of drug given, both tranquillisers and sedatives proved ineffective. The following day he gave the nurse who was attending him a series of notes saying, 'I am dying too slowly', 'Can someone please aid me very urgently?', 'Please give me very heavy doses of morphia plus calcium', 'How can I finish myself off please?', 'I am a doctor; this is genuine; I know I will obstruct again very soon – please help me', 'I am causing such misery to my wife, family and myself. Why do I have to go on with this useless pain?'.

These pleas were heart-rending enough, but they in no way express the terror and desperation in the man's eyes, each time he thrust another note into the nurse's hand. Eventually the medical staff agreed to increase the sedation until the patient lost consciousness. He died three days later.

It is hard to see what useful response could be expected from the nurse in this case. One thing she could do was to be with the patient for as much of the time as she possibly could. It was feasible on this occasion for the nurses to make out a rota. Each took their turn to sit with the patient for an hour at a time, so that he was never left alone. The other response was to keep the medical staff informed. This involved reporting back on the patient's condition every hour, until the nurses were satisfied that his suffering was being adequately relieved.

Every nurse and every doctor involved in this patient's care felt inadequate and anguished. The trust and respect which existed within the team was vital in enabling them to help the patient through his ordeal.

A great many nurses will, at some time in their working lives, wish that euthanasia were available for certain patients. But when one reflects on the implications of such legislation, it seems a daunting prospect. Who would authorise and give the fatal dose? Could we ensure that no one would die as a result of the emotional pressures created by its availability? How much guilt would be suffered by those who chose to live on? The questions are endless.

Wide agreement on this subject is very unlikely, because an individual's standpoint is dependent upon his philosophy and faith, on the value he places upon human life, and on his attitude towards human suffering. The status quo may in fact represent as close a compromise as is desirable or possible.

REFERENCE

Wilshaw, C., *The Right to Die*. British Humanist Association.

Chapter 11

Bereavement

Bereavement is the term used to describe the reaction to any major loss. Although its use is frequently confined to the after-effects of a death, it can be applied just as accurately to the reactions which may occur as the result of any other severe loss, such as retirement, redundancy, a broken marriage or the emigration of one's children. The same characteristics are also seen in the reaction to physical loss, such as an amputation, a mastectomy or failing eyesight.

When someone dies, all those whose lives were interwoven with that of the deceased will respond in some way. This will vary widely, in accordance with the depth and quality of the relationship that existed. It can range from a momentary feeling of sadness, to an overwhelming desolation which may persist for many years. Although usually predominant, grief is not the only emotion triggered by death. In some cases, it will produce nothing but pleasure and relief; more often it will arouse a whole spectrum of feelings.

The death of a spouse, a living companion or a child are amongst those losses likely to lead to the most intense form of grief. It is difficult to see the response to losing a toy, to a broken romance or to the death of a pet, for example, as being in any way connected with the raw grief of a parent whose child has recently died. However, all reactions to loss, from the most mild to the most profound, contain similar characteristics and require similar psychological coping mechanisms to deal with them. Consequently, previous experience of loss will have a strong bearing on the current response.

The intense grief which is likely to follow a death within the nuclear family, or that of a close friend, is the form of bereavement which nurses caring for the terminally ill encounter most often. This chapter concentrates largely upon the experiences and needs of people in this particular group.

LOSS OF LIFE-STYLE

The grief of bereavement is usually two-fold. There is not only the loss of the loved one but also, very often, the loss of a whole life-style. Death occurring prematurely will almost certainly have a great effect on the family income, possibly necessitating a move to a smaller house (and perhaps to a different area and a different school), or the mother who was previously a full-time housewife seeking paid employment outside of the home. Widowers with young children may find that they, too, have to change their work if it involves a great deal of travelling or arriving home late in the evenings. Many widows find themselves suddenly ostracised and their social life curtailed. This may be caused partly by the death taboo, but probably rather more by their new image as potential 'husband snatchers'.

The roles of older married couples tend to be very clearly defined, with minimal overlap. The practical dependency of one upon the other is therefore enormous, and many are incapable of an independent existence. A surprising number of newly bereaved widows have never paid a bill, signed a cheque, mown the lawn or driven the car, and a similarly large number of widowers have never washed a shirt, sewn a button on or cooked a meal. The death of someone who has previously cared for a disabled relative, can leave the latter unable to remain in his own home. Coping with the move into an institution whilst grieving over the loss of a loved one, the loss of a home and a whole way of life, must be one of the most intolerable forms bereavement can take.

PSYCHOLOGICAL ADAPTATION

Although the grief of bereavement may cause such desolation in the first weeks and months after a death, most people are then able to mobilise their coping mechanisms and work through a process of adaptation, until they eventually reach a resolution of their grief. The emotions and psychological stages through which they are likely to pass bear a strong resemblance to those experienced by the dying patient. The omission of one or more of the stages and the to-ing and fro-ing, the progressing and regressing, are also similar.

When young children are parted from their parents for a prolonged period, they have been seen to pass through a series of emotions in adapting to their new situation. This turmoil is known as 'separation anxiety'. They look around frantically, trying to locate their parents;

they scream with rage when they realise that they have been deserted; they pine longingly for their return, then sink into a state of apathy, sadness and withdrawal. Eventually, they adapt and start to relate to new, substitute parents, but their ability to trust and establish close relationships may never totally recover. In following the bereaved person through their process of adaptation, it is interesting to note how closely it relates to the separation anxiety of children.

SHOCK

The first stage, as with the person facing death, is shock. It presents in one of the same two ways, panic or numbness, and may last from a few minutes to a few days. The bereaved person, with the hyperactivity of panic, may rush around arranging the funeral single-handed and may even start sorting out the deceased person's possessions on the day of his death, but show no evidence of grieving. In complete contrast is the numbed, apathetic person, whose family and friends will have to take on all the necessary arrangements and even perform essential household tasks for him.

Shock reactions defend us from the first full impact of what has happened. Pangs of acute grief, which feel almost identical to fear, pierce their way with increasing frequency through this blanket of shock, until its protective covering is completely destroyed. The bereaved person is now at his most vulnerable, completely exposed to the pain of grieving. Other defence mechanisms will frequently take over, but sooner or later this grief will re-emerge. Not until it has been suffered in all its depth, intensity and length will it recede, allowing resolution to occur. There is no easy escape route.

If the death is expected and prepared for emotionally, the grieving will already have begun. Although this does not mean that the pain is any less, it does mean that the element of shock is reduced and the grieving is usually less turbulent as a result.

ACUTE GRIEF

The physiological changes experienced, when in the throes of acute grief, are brought about by stimulation of the sympathetic nervous system and the inhibition of the parasympathetic. This is the same 'fight and flight' response which is also produced by fear, pain and anger. The grieving person is in a state of high arousal, and muscular tension, insomnia and anorexia are common.

There is usually a great feeling of restlessness, moving about aimlessly, searching for something to do. Whilst in this state of agitation and arousal, the bereaved person constantly pines for the one who has died. Preoccupation with thoughts of the lost person and the events leading up to their death usually result in intermittent periods of crying, and an inability to concentrate on anything else. The ability to function adequately at home, at school or at work is greatly diminished. Although thinking about the lost person is guaranteed to produce pain, the compulsion to do so makes it irresistible.

But acute grief is not normally experienced continuously for more than a few weeks. Although the high arousal and restlessness may continue, gradually increasing periods of time will elapse between thinking about and longing for the dead person. Within a month or two, most people find themselves able to function reasonably well again, despite the pangs of grief which sometimes grip them. Only when the demands of the day have been met do they allow themselves time to weep and mourn again.

DENIAL AND SEARCHING

The next stage is one of denial of the death and searching for the deceased person. This may take the form of a spiritual quest. Because the 'life-force' of the person who died had such a profound effect upon the person who is left, the latter may find it impossible to accept that this could simply have been extinguished. Consequently, they search in their minds for the answer as to where the 'life-force' or spirit has gone. This may even result in a conversion to a new faith. Quite apart from the inability to believe that the death of a loved one can possibly mean their total extinction, any belief in some form of after-life also carries with it the most comforting of all possibilities, that of a future reunion with the deceased.

During this period of denial of the finality of death and searching for the present spiritual whereabouts of the loved one, long periods of time may be spent in daydreaming about the way in which future meetings with the deceased will occur. Even those with no real belief in a future meeting may gain comfort from imagining what it would be like if their loved one were to come back for just a few hours. Some will be so determined in their denial of death's finality that they may visit spiritualists in the hope of being put into communication with the deceased.

There may even be a search for the physical whereabouts of the person who has died, but this is an unusual mental state. Those who enter it may get 'stuck' and require psychiatric help to move on. This is demonstrated by the following quotations which were taken from four letters written by a widower during the first year after his wife's death. She died suddenly and unexpectedly, after many years of suffering from a degenerative neurological disease.

'. . . Dear Sister, I write this because I am so terribly lonely and fed up. I have been here all of Saturday and today and the emptiness is enough to send one round the bend. Another reason I send this is that, although there is a grave here and my Rose is supposed to be there, I have a terrible job believing this. You see, when I sit and think, the last time I saw Rose, She was in bed and although She did not speak and I was very upset, I often wonder if She was only in a very deep sleep. These thoughts lead me to think that my Rose is still in the hospital and I am not allowed to see Her.

There is hardly a day goes by that I do not go to the hospital, ride round hoping I am going to see my Rose. It does not matter how much I try not to come near the hospital, I just ride round and suddenly I find myself in the hospital again. So often I would have liked to have come in . . .'

'. . . I can honestly say at times I feel that no one would mind if I were not here any more. The only reason I have not done something before now is that I feel Rose will be back and She would not be happy on Her own and there would be no one to take care of Her. So I sit and wait, for I know that as soon as She is well again She will let me know where I can find Her.

I feel there is not much use in anything now without my Rose. She was my life and until I can find Her, I think things will not change. Every day seems longer and more lonely and at times I get the feeling that people are watching me and saying things I cannot hear. Then I get to thinking they know something they will not tell me.

I know I need help but I don't know what kind. If I see the doctor, I only get told it will pass and get more pills. Please forgive me for I must do something, always hoping someone will put me on the right track . . .'

'. . . I do not feel well and I am so lonely that at times I get to thinking that it is no good to keep trying. Things do not get better and the more I try, the more I miss my Rose. I can hear Her talking much more now. At times Her talking and knocking on the wall makes the dog bark and she rushes into the bedroom. I feel sure that if something doesn't get me out of this mess soon I shall do something silly, I am getting much more depressed all the time . . .'

'. . . I thought that as the time passed I would be getting over the loss, but I find myself missing Her more and I still keep thinking She is in the hospital, only I can't find out where. I doze off to sleep and I can see Her there in that bed, and I get to thinking my Rose was only in a very deep sleep because of the drugs. Also, every now and then I hear Her calling my name. When I wake I feel I want to go to Her, but I do not know where to go . . .'

Despite frequent visits to the hospital throughout this year, regular bereavement counselling sessions and, on one occasion, looking into every room, office and cupboard, it was impossible to help this man for a very long time. In fact it was three years before the first signs of recovery were seen. Although bereavement counselling is not an area in which to expect easy or speedy solutions, this was an unusually protracted case.

PRETENCE OR FANTASY

The next possible stage that bereaved people may enter is pretence or fantasy. This is when one finds someone cooking a meal, intentionally, for the deceased person, laying out his clothes ready for him to wear that day, warming his slippers and holding imaginary conversations. This is not to be confused with the widow who, having laid the table for two people for forty years, finds herself occasionally forgetting and laying her husband's place. Nor is it to be confused with the person who converses either silently or aloud with the deceased person, fully aware that he is dead. This is not pretence; it is an intentional way of obtaining support from the deceased person's memory. Particularly when a decision of the type always previously made by the spouse is required, the widowed person frequently acts out a conversation to help himself imagine what advice the deceased person would have given. Most newly bereaved people have a very strong sense of the presence of the person who has died. This again is not fantasy, but a very real feeling or even a hallucination. Pretence or fantasy occurs when a person is unable to or refuses to come to terms with the reality of the death. The finality, the guilt, the pain and the loneliness are too much to accept, so he escapes into a world of make-believe.

GUILT

The quality of a relationship before someone dies is largely responsible for the quality of the bereavement. A deeply loving and long-lasting relationship can result in complete anguish and desolation, the pain of which is indescribable. However, love of this quality seems to enable the healing process to take place. Although the pain of the loss is so great, the strength of the love which has been shared often seems to carry the bereaved person through to a resolution of their grief. In a relationship where there has been a lot of distrust, bitterness and pain, there may be a large element of relief at the death. In some cases, where the degree of pain has far outweighed any happiness the relationship may have given, particularly if the deceased person was largely responsible, relief may be the predominant feeling. Many previously oppressed husbands and wives take on a new lease of life and experience some of their happiest and most fulfilled years during widowhood. However, the negative element in most relationships is fairly reciprocal. Consequently, guilt at the pain caused to the deceased, plus guilt at the feelings of relief at their death, will be more common. It is this guilt which prolongs and distorts so many bereavements. The bereft person is constantly trying to dispel the guilt both from his own mind and from the minds of others. He frequently idealises the deceased person and their relationship. It will seem ridiculous to close friends and relatives, hearing the person who has previously only ever been described in the most derisory of terms, now being raised above the human race to a pedestal of inimitable perfection. The following letter was from a widow whose marriage had been full of unhappiness. When the deceased was diagnosed, his wife was living with her brother, having left her husband six months previously. However, when the time came that he needed help in the home and, later on, in nursing care, she returned to look after him.

'. . . Thank you so much for all that you did for my dear Herbert during his last days. He was so brave through all those months of terrible suffering. Even while he was so ill he never even complained – always worrying about all the work he was making for me and worrying about how I'd manage after he'd passed away.

I really don't know how I'm going to live without him. We had twenty-two perfect years together – never a cross word spoken between us. Everyone always said how much he adored me – no husband could have been more generous than he was, nothing was too much trouble or too expensive for me. And we shared everything, we never kept any secrets or worries from one another.

We gave him a funeral service fit for a king – no more than he deserved though. We had a full choir and there were flowers on every window ledge of the church. I laid on a buffet lunch for fifty afterwards, with waitresses and the lot.

I've just been to the grave to put some fresh flowers on it. There's so much to do sorting out all his clothes and everything . . .'

The only way forward in a case such as this is for the bereaved person to be helped to acknowledge and accept the causes of their guilt.

Many bereaved people chastise themselves about their own inadequacy in caring for the dying person. If hospital admission was necessitated, this may be surrounded by irrational guilt. Thoughts about the possibility of an earlier diagnosis having procured a cure will also be a source of guilt. Convictions that they were impatient, unloving and lacking in warmth and affection will be another. There may be a need for constant and repeated reassurances on all these issues for many months.

ANGER

Anger is one of our most primitive and forceful emotions. It is not surprising, therefore, that its expression in bereavement seems childlike and irrational. Great waves of it sweep over the unsuspecting person, filling him with bitterness and resentment towards the deceased for having died and caused him so much pain, for leaving him alone to cope with three young children, or for not fighting harder against the disease. He may be angry with God or with fate, especially if the death was premature, and he may be angry with the doctors and nursing staff, which need or need not be rational. Relatives, friends and neighbours are also likely targets, as the bereaved person frequently feels that the amount of time, support and practical help received, both before and after the death, was less than it should have been.

If this anger can be vented and accepted as perfectly normal, and not as a cause for guilt and shame, it will gradually subside. While it lasts, its expression can be a valuable means of relieving accumulated stress. Occasionally, anger will be a means of expressing grief, particularly in the male who links masculinity with the 'stiff upper lip'. This was demonstrated by a young man whose wife had just had a stillborn baby. On visiting their home, the wife was found to be, quite naturally, overwhelmed with grief and crying continuously. The husband, meanwhile, was stamping around the house making terrible, unfounded accusations against both the doctor and the midwife. His anger made him quite unable to hear any rational explanation of the true cause of the tragedy, or to share in his wife's grieving and offer her any support.

The visitor suggested he should pretend that she was the midwife concerned and that he should tell her exactly what he would like to say if she were really there. An incredible flow of abuse and display of anger ensued, lasting for between five and ten minutes. Although there was embarrassment at first, he became increasingly uninhibited and heated. Quite suddenly the outburst ceased, and the bereft father was shaking with great sobs of grief. When the visitor left, husband and wife were crying in each other's arms, consoling each other by the sharing of their sorrow.

DEPRESSION

As the months since the death begin to pass, the acute pain of grief is gradually replaced by a dull ache, often experienced as a period of depression. Uncertainty, apathy and despondency are common features. Many of the bereaved will now withdraw from society, lacking the necessary confidence to relate to strangers or casual acquaintances. Unless forced to do otherwise by circumstances, such as the need to earn a living, there is a tendency to spend a great deal of time with close friends and relatives with whom the bereaved person feels protected, cared for and unthreatened. Anorexia, insomnia and a lack of energy are usual, the latter often resulting in long periods of time being spent alone and inactive. The severely depressed seem unable to cope with life. Absenteeism from work is common and there may be a dramatic fall in standards, both in personal appearance as well as in the upkeep of the home and garden.

Spending time with someone who is depressed offers little reward. Consequently, they are in danger of becoming alienated and isolated. This in turn reinforces the depression. Amongst those referred for psychiatric help during bereavement, by far the greatest proportion present with depression.

LONELINESS

Loneliness is a large part of all bereavement, desperately missing being with the person who has died. But the loneliness of those left to live alone after many years of sharing their home and life with another person must be the worst loneliness of all. Life can seem completely empty: getting up alone, planning one's day alone, shopping for oneself, cooking for oneself, no one to share the snippets of gossip or the interesting newspaper articles with, long silent evenings which end in going to bed alone, the latter being the worst time of all.

This is a normal and acceptable pattern of living for many single people, but to the newly bereaved the unfamiliarity of the loneliness heightens the feeling of desolation. The majority of middle-aged or elderly people have never lived alone before widowhood, having moved straight from their family home into their married home. The adjustment they must make to cope with this new life style is colossal. It is not surprising that many hardly attempt it, preferring to relinquish their own homes and live with a relative, or even to re-marry within a matter of months.

Isolation of this nature, following a death, is inevitable in a society where each nuclear family lives in its own unit of accommodation, usually separated by many miles from the extended family. The bereaved can be seen to adjust far more easily in other societies where this is not the case, and where loneliness is not nearly such a dominant feature.

Of course, not only married people live in couples and run the risk of being left to live a solitary existence following the death of their partner; homosexual couples, friends, siblings and the unmarried sons or daughters who live with a widowed or single parent all run the same risk. There is an additional component to the loneliness experienced on the loss of a sexual partner. Just at the time when physical closeness and warmth is most needed to ease the pain of grief, that comfort is denied the bereaved person. This can lead to an intense longing for sexual contact and not infrequently to a greatly increased libido. This may be suppressed, or it may be acted upon, but either way it is likely to lead to feelings of shame and guilt at the lack of loyalty and love shown for the deceased. This guilt will almost certainly be reinforced by family or friends should the bereaved person decide to confide in them. The possibility of this increased sexual desire should be borne in mind by those offering counselling and emotional support to the newly bereaved.

The death of someone who has required constant attention for a long period of time, such as a severely handicapped child who lives into his teens, or an adult who has a prolonged neurological disease, will leave the person who has cared for him especially lonely. Their whole life has often revolved around caring for the sick person for so long that all other interests, activities and friends have been forced into the background, leaving a complete void when he dies.

RESOLUTION

The final stage of bereavement is that of resolution. This does not mean a cessation of love for, or memories about, the person who has died, or even an end to the pain of missing them. What it does mean is that the grief and other distressing feelings have been worked through sufficiently to allow the bereaved person to function at their previous level again, to have positive feelings about their life and future, and to begin to develop the trust required to form new relationships. The amount of time it takes to reach this stage can vary from about six months to never. The most common time interval is probably about two years, but the older the person and the longer their relationship has endured, the longer it generally takes.

As people grow older they find it increasingly difficult to adjust to change, particularly in their own daily routine. Those with any degree of senile dementia find it even harder to cope with. The death of a living companion will be more than many elderly people are ever able to adjust to, and many will continue to grieve until they die themselves.

Every geriatric ward will have its quota of demented, widowed patients, who almost daily work through a programme of one minute asking for their spouse, as though thinking they are still alive, and the next minute weeping tears of grief at their death. However much loving support is given, they will probably still be expressing their grief in an identical manner many years later, apparently quite incapable of progressing towards any resolution of their feelings.

During bereavement, a number of people go through a process of introjection. This is the absorption of skills, interests and mannerisms of the deceased person into the personality of the one who is left. It occurs to some extent in nearly all marriages or partnerships, without anyone dying, but the speed at which so many facets of the partner's personality can be acquired during bereavement is quite startling. This process does not seem to be detrimental to the resolution of grief. It may in fact make letting go of the past easier, as there is no danger of forgetting or losing something that has become a part of oneself.

If a bereaved person was able to talk openly to their loved one during the months before the death occurred, and they were able to make plans and decisions for the future jointly, it will provide a tremendous source of strength and comfort during the early months of bereavement as well as fostering a positive attitude towards the future.

As previously stated, those who are able to work through to a resolution of their grief continue to feel great sadness at their loss. So much more tolerable is this than the earlier pain, however, that they frequently think that their grief is 'cured', and are then overwhelmed with despair when a television programme or a chance meeting with an old friend evokes a pang of grief with all the intensity of earlier days. They need to be prepared for these recurrences, especially on their own or the deceased person's birthday, on their wedding anniversary, Christmas, or the anniversary of the death.

So the pain of loss will never disappear completely, but many people are able to grow as a result of their suffering, in a way they never could have done without it.

HELPING THE MOURNING PROCESS

RITUALS

Immediately following a death, the ritualistic activities of viewing the body, arranging the funeral and receiving the condolences create a framework within which the bereaved person feels he has the permission and safety to mourn the loss of his loved one. If they were not with the deceased person at the time of death, viewing the body may be vital to remove any doubts that they might still be alive. In addition, it creates an opportunity for saying 'goodbye'. The very changed appearance of the body will help the bereaved to begin to face up to the reality of death. The corpse looks so obviously like a shell from which the person has departed.

Nurses have a responsibility for encouraging this activity as a means of enabling the grieving process to begin as early as possible. This may involve the firm handling of friends and relatives who frequently try to dissuade the bereaved person from spending time with the body. This will invariably arise from their concern to protect them from any unnecessary pain, but the nurse should help them to understand that the pain is inevitable, and that the earlier this grieving process begins, the less likely it is to be distorted or protracted.

There is considerable pressure in our 'death-denying' society to abandon all the rituals surrounding a death. We no longer have the body lying at home, we rarely wear black, letters of condolence are reduced to pre-printed cards, and even the traditional flowers and wreaths are fast losing popularity. There may be quite justifiable reasons for not throwing away large sums of money on flowers, but we should be aware of these pressures and ensure that sufficient ritual is retained to encourage the mourning process. We have much to learn in this respect from both Eastern and Latin cultures, where the body is still kept at home so that the family, friends and neighbours can care for it and pay their last respects. Funeral wakes are much more prevalent, and the whole procedure is likely to be more participatory and free from anonymity than in the West. Displays of grieving are not treated as something to be ashamed of or to be ignored by embarrassed bystanders.

BEREAVEMENT COUNSELLING

Within a few days of the funeral, the extended family will once more have dispersed to their various corners of the earth and the upsurge of neighbourliness will have subsided. Families have a great tendency to swamp the bereaved person with support immediately following the death and then to withdraw completely. It is so much more helpful when the time given in the early days is limited, but a regular commitment to visiting is planned over the ensuing months. Unless this happens, the bereaved person may become dependent on voluntary and statutory bodies to provide the care and support which they are sure to need, and this is increasingly the case.

Bereavement is a time when people tend to shy away. Their own fears of death and their embarrassment at any display of grief may prevent them from offering companionship and care. It is sad to see the need for 'outside' help in this area increasing, but it is certainly necessary, since few peoplé can survive bereavement without some sort of help. Voluntary organisations such as the Samaritans and Cruse are now training counsellors to meet this need, and health visitors, community nurses, general practitioners and social workers increasingly regard it as part of their work. The sad thing is the apparent decline in the amount of support given by family, friends and colleagues. However, the increased understanding of bereavement by the various groups of caring professionals, and their recognition of the needs it creates, is encouraging.

THE ROLE OF THE NURSE-COUNSELLOR

The nurse who has helped care for a dying patient at home is in an ideal position to offer support during bereavement, if she feels that this is needed. However, it must be realised at the outset that a great deal of time and motivation is required, and an honest admission to herself that she lacks either or both of these is perfectly acceptable. The one thing that is not acceptable is a half-hearted approach, particularly when the bereaved person is allowed to develop a dependency on the nurse, only to have the visits curtailed while still in the acute stage of grieving. Many community nurses make a habit of paying just one bereavement visit. This is usually during the week of the death, and is often the time when loaned nursing equipment and left-over drugs are collected. Even a 'one-off' visit of this kind can be very supportive, without giving the relative any false hopes of a continuing relationship.

The alternative is a commitment to regular, lengthy visits, when a counselling model is adopted (see page 56). Since time is always in short supply, it may be appropriate to offer this kind of help only to those people who seem to be in the greatest need. These will include the ones who refused to accept that death was imminent; those for whom the death came suddenly, with no prior warning; those who had an abnormal response to the death or no response at all; those with a history of psychiatric illness, particularly depression; those with no friends or relatives with whom they have a close, supportive relationship; the elderly, particularly the physically frail or those with mental impairment, who are left to live alone; and those who are left single-handed to care for a young family.

The prime task of the counsellor is to enable the bereaved person to talk about the one who has died, about his life, his personality, his illness and death, and about their relationship. Express 'permission' may be needed to reassure the client that this is acceptable to the counsellor, since they may already have attempted similar sharing with friends and found the conversation rapidly diverted onto more cheerful matters. The friends may well have thought that they were acting in the best interest of the bereaved person, protecting them from a conversation which was sure to arouse painful feelings, as well as protecting themselves. But the thoughts and feelings will be there just the same, and most people feel a strong need to share them. The simplest way for the nurse-counsellor to give this 'permission' is to initiate a conversation about the deceased person herself.

Grief, anger, relief and guilt are the feelings most likely to be expressed. Crying should be possible without any loss of self-respect; in fact tears should be welcomed. Physical contact, in the form of an arm around the shoulder, holding a hand, or even a hug, may increase the safety which is necessary to enable the sharing of painful thoughts and feelings. This will require great sensitivity, however, as some people would be distressed by such unfamiliar intimacy, particularly if client and counsellor were of the opposite sex.

Grieving can be seen as the job which every bereaved person must undertake. Tackling painful feelings is extremely hard work, and it is not surprising that many people try every possible tactic to avoid doing so. The counsellor will need to encourage her clients in their work, avoiding the temptation to slip into superficial chatter. Accounts of particularly distressing events will need to be recalled again and again.

GUILT

Where guilt is a predominant feature, the nurse is often in a good position to help alleviate it. She may be able to assure the bereaved person that an earlier diagnosis would not have affected the outcome of the illness. She can usually validate their care of the dying person, giving assurances that he felt much loved and was always given the very best of care. Nevertheless, there will be times when this is not possible. Those who did not allow the dying person to talk openly with them about their situation, those who behaved unlovingly or those who never attempted to get their wife to a doctor, despite their awareness of a growing breast lump, for example, are amongst the ones for whom hollow reassurances would be meaningless. The presence of the counsellor will often make the guilt feelings seem less threatening, and her help in exploring the causes of unloving behaviour may produce answers which will lessen the pain.

DREAMS

One of the most common causes of anxiety in early bereavement is the nature and content of dreams. These are frequently about the deceased person and are particularly vivid and realistic. It seems strange that people should expect all trace of their loved ones to be immediately erased from their dreams when they die, but this is very often the case. Many people are convinced that they are becoming insane because of the presence of the deceased in their dreams. Others are alarmed by strange tales of reincarnation and resurrection experienced during their sleep; these take many forms, but always involve the bringing back to life of the deceased. It is important to remember to ask the bereaved person if they are experiencing any strange dreams, for they are often too afraid or ashamed to volunteer the information without prompting. If they are, their normality must be emphasised repeatedly.

PRETENCE AND FANTASY

If there is any pretence or fantasy that the deceased person is still alive, or any searching for his physical whereabouts, the bereaved person will frequently experience brief flashes of insight into his own bizarre behaviour. Again, the primary need is for constant reassurance that this behaviour is typical and normal.

SUICIDAL THOUGHTS

It is hardly surprising that many of the bereaved wish at some point that they too were dead, or that this longing is translated into suicidal thoughts. The counsellor may sometimes fear that this is the case but be unsure how to help, since no such thoughts have been verbalised. One solution is to wait until the client is next expressing feelings of grief, when it may seem quite appropriate to enquire whether or not it has ever felt so awful that he has contemplated ending his own life. It is most unlikely that this approach would ever encourage a suicide attempt, but it may well help to avoid one. By being bold enough to raise such a taboo subject, the counsellor may find that she has enabled the bereaved person to share thoughts which would otherwise have seemed too terrifying and shameful to reveal.

If, at the end of the counselling session, the client is still expressing determination to take his own life, the general practitioner should be consulted. It is to be hoped that he will make an urgent visit, and possibly offer to refer them to a psychiatrist, although this will not always be the answer. It is important that the counsellor continues to think clearly and avoids panicking. She may well be able to discover ways in which the life of the bereaved person can be made a little more bearable. If loneliness is a problem, it may be possible for the counsellor to take them to a meeting of Cruse, to obtain help from the church community or to enlist the support of neighbours, for example, always with the client's prior permission. If lack of sleep has been a problem, the doctor may prescribe a sedative, or if they are experiencing panic attacks, an anxiolytic drug. However, the danger of leaving a suicidal person with large quantities of drugs that depress the central nervous system must also be borne in mind.

Sometimes nothing seems to help. The return of the dead person is the only thing that will make life worth living again, and this no one can bring about. If the determination to commit suicide is great enough, even the most skilful counsellor or psychotherapist will sometimes fail to prevent it.

REVISITING OLD HAUNTS

Most families and friends have places which they visit together often and which have particular significance for them. This may be a favourite walk or picnic spot, a restaurant or holiday home. Revisiting these places for the first time, without the person who has died, can be a poignant or much-feared experience. The longer it is delayed, the worse is the suffering, as the pain of anticipation can be as severe as the actual pain of the event.

The bereavement counsellor should ask if there are such places and offer to accompany the bereaved person on any such outing. They may prefer to go alone, in which case the offer of a visit on their return may be helpful.

If the deceased person was in hospital for any length of time before the death occurred, this may be the place which holds the most vivid and painful memories, and the place which is hardest to revisit. Until they have entered the hospital again and spoken with the staff who cared for the deceased during his last weeks, the compulsion to do so may hang over the bereaved person, filling them with anxiety and dread. A warm invitation from the hospital staff to revisit the ward at any time can so easily be given when handing over the death certificate, and will make the revisiting far easier. If this invitation is followed up, it is vital that a warm welcome is given, even though the relative is sure to arrive at the most hectic and inconvenient moment. Pre-arranged appointments may be essential on some acute wards.

MAJOR DECISIONS

In order to escape from the pain of grieving, many people will make major decisions within the first six months of the death. These frequently include moving house in order to escape from the memories. The memories are of course not dissipated by the move, and as the grief begins to resolve, the loss of a dearly loved family home may be a source of great regret. However, family homes are frequently impractical and not financially viable for a widowed person, and too long a delay in making the decision to move may well result in their staying permanently in an unsuitable home. If a hasty move is unavoidable, every attempt should be made to persuade the bereaved person to stay in the same, familiar neighbourhood.

Another decision, also frequently taken too soon and which has already been mentioned briefly, is the decision to re-marry. Widowers fall into this trap far more often than widows. Even in the elderly, when marriage is embarked upon explicitly for the sake of companionship, unhappiness may well result. The bereaved person will either suppress his need to grieve, which may well result in all manner of physical and emotional ailments, or else he will go ahead and mourn his loved one, in which case he will be quite oblivious to the emotional needs of his new spouse. Adjustment to a new living partner is always demanding and is just not compatible with the emotional cost of grieving.

For similar reasons, many people will change their jobs in an attempt to leave their pain behind, to start a completely new life with others who know nothing of their past suffering. As must be clear by now, however firmly it is suppressed, grief will surface eventually in one form or another. The ease with which a familiar job can be handled, and the comfort of familiar colleagues who understand the pain which is being endured, will be a far better environment for the newly bereaved person than the unfamiliarity and challenge of a new job.

When young children die, parents will often rush into having another baby, thinking that it will replace the one who has died and so remove the pain of grief. Of course this is never the case, and many parents later regret their decision. As the new baby develops, every stage produces poignant memories of their dead child, and the grief that these memories evoke may inhibit the nurturing of their 'replacement child'.

One final decision which may be made too hastily is the decision to dispose of every possession previously owned by the deceased. Once more, the reasoning behind it is to escape from painful memories. And once more, the reasoning behind discouraging such a decision is the necessity and unavoidability of grieving. As with the family home, which is lost for ever, tremendous regret at the loss of possessions much loved by the deceased is sure to follow. When the grieving begins to resolve, few things can give greater pleasure and evoke happier memories than these objects. The other end of this spectrum is the widow who keeps every item of her husband's clothing untouched in the drawers and cupboards. This may be due to denial of the death and will hinder the possibility of resolving the grief.

The role of the nurse-counsellor in this situation is to discourage hasty decision-making on any major issues during the first few months of bereavement, delaying them for two years, whenever practicable.

DANGER SIGNALS

Bereavement is not an illness, but a healthy reaction to loss. However, some people do become either physically or psychiatrically ill, or both, during their bereavement. The groups of people most at risk are the same as those cited as being in greatest need of bereavement counselling (see page 224). There are several danger signals which indicate that grief is not following a normal pattern and may become pathological. The first of these is a complete lack of response to the death; the bereaved person behaves as though he has not comprehended when told that the death has occurred, and the acute stage of grieving is either delayed, or in some cases omitted altogether. The second indicator is a prolonged state of shock, lasting for several days or even weeks. The third is a prolongation of acute grieving. This stage, when crying is common and pining for the deceased is almost constant, normally lasts for only a few weeks. The fourth and final indicator is an excessive degree of guilt and remorse.

If these danger signals are not picked up and there is no early intervention, the bereaved person may present later with one or more of a wide range of conditions, of which by far the most common is severe and protracted depression. All the manifestations of pathological grief, including depression, are the same as those seen in normal patterns of grieving, the difference being their severity and duration. Apart from depression, small numbers of patients will present with alcoholism, phobic symptoms or panic attacks and, very rarely, in a psychotic condition with hallucinations and delusions. Physical conditions related to stress, such as headaches, asthma, colitis and dyspepsia, are common: coronary artery disease is another, which probably gave rise to the saying 'dying from a broken heart'. Hypochondriacal symptoms, otherwise known as conversion-hysteria, are also prevalent, frequently mimicking the symptoms of the deceased.

The nurse-counsellor will soon learn to recognise pathological grieving, and her response should always be to seek the backing of the general practitioner, who may decide that psychiatric referral is warranted. Too liberal a prescription of sedatives and tranquillisers is an accusation frequently aimed at general practitioners. But there is no way that they can allocate sufficient time to meet the need for bereavement counselling themselves, with the work pressure as it now stands, hence the need for more health visitors, community nurses and voluntary counselling services to take on this task. Sedatives do have a use, of course, particularly when the dead person has been cared for at home and sleep has been disturbed for many weeks. One week's supply of a night sedative, halving the dose for the last two or three nights, may be all that is necessary to re-establish the sleep pattern. Repeat prescriptions should not be given without a thorough review of the case.

COMPANIONSHIP

Quite apart from specific counselling, the bereaved person will have an enormous need for companionship, although invitations to noisy parties or similar frivolities will be neither helpful nor appropriate in the early months. Any encouragement to 'snap out of it' and act as though nothing has happened will merely succeed in encouraging the suppression of grief. However, invitations to join friends for a meal, a walk, a picnic, a quiet drink or to come and stay for a few days, will be invaluable. But these must be accompanied by an awareness of the need for solitude, since some grieving can only be done at home, alone. The desire for solitude, or fear of it, will vary widely.

An early morning telephone call from a friend can make all the difference to a day in which the bereaved person might otherwise have convinced himself that nobody cared whether he was dead or alive. In the middle of the night, wandering around an empty house, feelings of panic, fear and grief can seem at their most threatening and intolerable. A telephone call to a friend or counsellor who has specifically asked to be called in such an event can be a valuable safety valve.

When the acute stage of bereavement begins to pass and the times of weeping and despair are coming less frequently, gentle encouragement will be required to renew old interests and take up new ones, to get out and about again and make new friends. There may be some diffidence about this, stemming from fear of being disloyal to the deceased and the fear that others may assume that they have already forgotten about their loved one. There may be a lack of confidence caused by the change in marital status, since this is often experienced as a loss of status. If this kind of encouragement is given too early, it will be interpreted as a lack of understanding of the true depth of the grief.

The anniversary of the death is, for many people, just as painful a time as the time of the death itself. Letters of sympathy and visits can help greatly. Perhaps the most important way of helping is by writing or talking about the deceased. The bereaved person will have absorbed by now the full impact of the reality and finality of the death. He will feel isolated, imagining that he alone remembers the loved one. It will give enormous comfort to share memories of the past with friends and relatives.

Those who have lost a living companion will need to acquire a vast range of new skills. These will range from car maintenance, paying the bills and home decorating to sewing, gardening and housewifery. For those who find it easier to give more practical forms of help, this is a perfect opening.

CHILDREN

Children who lose someone close to them, especially a parent or sibling, are rarely given adequate support. There are many reasons for this. The adult from whom they need support will almost certainly be suffering from acute grief himself, and will find it easy to justify the lack of explanations and support given to the child.

Under about nine years of age, few children are able to comprehend the full meaning and gravity of death. Their egotism frequently makes them feel that they are responsible for the death, either by having been angry with the deceased or by some other naughtiness for which this is now the punishment. However, they do not understand the finality, and will fully expect the deceased to revive and return. For this reason, death will evoke no greater emotional response than a temporary separation, and total absorption and enjoyment in play on the very day of the death can make this blatantly obvious. But the young child is acutely aware of the grief of other family members, and this will have a profound effect on him. A widowed mother, overwhelmed by grief (whether displayed before the child or concealed) and obliged to take a job for financial reasons, will have far less time and far less emotional energy for her children than she used to. This may have a far more serious and long-lasting effect on the child than the death itself.

Despite their lack of comprehension, young children do require some explanation when someone close to them is dying or has died. Only by honest explanation can the child be relieved of his sense of guilt about the cause of the death, and make some sense of the emotional turmoil going on around him. He, too, will need to work through his bereavement, often in games, fantasy, painting or making up stories.

The insecurity he experiences, both as a result of the deceased person being missing and the grieving going on around him, will lead to an increased need for cuddles and an unwillingness to be alone. Nightmares and regressive behaviour are also very common.

If there has previously been any attempt to explain the meaning of death to a child, it will certainly be rewarded. If he has experienced the death of a pet, an insect or a bird, and has been allowed to spend time observing how different a dead creature is from one that is alive, it may well obviate the need to answer such impossible questions as 'Where has Mummy gone now she's dead?' Many of the traditional replies, such as 'She's gone to be with Jesus' or 'She's gone to heaven' can lead to all kinds of confused thinking in a young child, especially if they are led to believe that she went away from choice.

Children over nine years old can begin to understand the full implications of death, and their mourning will be a mixture of some of the components of the younger child's process and some of those seen in adult grieving. Fits of crying, aggressive outbursts, or withdrawal and apathy are all common. The parent who can swallow his adult pride and share his grief with his child, weeping together, will both gain and give an enormous amount of support.

The older child or adolescent, whose grieving follows much the same pattern as an adult, often feels angry and hurt about the way his role is perceived. When a parent or sibling has died, his grief may receive little consideration, being seen as subsidiary to the parent's grief. When a parent of the same sex has died, children are frequently told by well-meaning adults that now their job is to assume the role of the dead person and to take care of their remaining parent. They may hear their parent being told to keep going for the sake of the children, or they may find themselves sent away for a holiday, to relieve the burden on their grieving parent.

All of these messages can increase the pain of the young person, because each one expresses concern for the parent's grief and each ignores the importance and depth of his own. He may feel that his love for the dead parent or sibling was greater than anyone else's, and also his feeling of loss. It is vital that the grief of young people is treated with the full concern and respect it deserves. There are no grounds for assuming that their capacity for love or grief is any less than that of an adult. Individual letters of condolence will mean so much more to an older child than one to the whole family.

REFERENCES

Murray Parkes, C., *Bereavement*. Penguin, 1972.
Wolffe, Sula, *Children Under Stress*. Penguin, 1973.

Chapter 12

The Needs of the Nursing Team

The team involved in the care of a dying patient at home usually consists of family members, friends and neighbours, plus the primary health care team. In many cases, it may also include a home help, a night sitter, a minister of religion and a social worker. Should admission to hospital be necessary, the list will more than double, largely due to the increase in the number of nurses involved. This is, of course, one of the arguments for keeping patients at home whenever possible, where continuity and depth in relationships with the nursing staff is more feasible.

Attending to the needs of the patient's family and loved ones is an integral part of caring for the dying person. As such, it has been described in the course of this book, and the following account therefore concentrates on the needs of a nursing team involved in the care of the dying, though their needs will differ little from their colleagues in other professions.

Each member of the team has needs which are dependent upon their degree of involvement with the patient, their previous experience with those who are dying, and their own feelings about death. Those who have had a recent bereavement themselves and those who have unresolved grief will need additional support to deal with their own feelings, which are sure to be restimulated by both the patient and his family. When caring for cancer patients, those who have had any form of cancer themselves will also need extra support to cope with the resurgence of fears about the possibility of their disease recurring and even of their own death.

Every member of the team is a unique person with a unique set of needs, just as is the case with patients and relatives. It is still not uncommon to find amongst the caring professions an attitude of indifference towards the feelings of members of staff. The commitment to self-sacrifice lingers on, with any concern for one's own feelings, or those of one's colleagues, being regarded as self-indulgent. There is no doubt that, to care for a dying person effectively, a certain amount of self-sacrifice is unavoidable. However, it is only when this is accompanied by recognition and acceptance of one's own feelings that the channels of communication offering effective sharing and support are opened. It is part of the responsibility of every member of the nursing team to be aware of both her own and her colleagues' feelings and needs, doing all within her scope to meet them.

INTERDEPENDENCE

When considering the needs of a team, there are certain principles which should be taken into account. These apply equally to a team on a car assembly line and a team caring for terminally ill patients. Effective functioning depends on three major factors. The first is the achievement of the task, in this case providing the highest possible standard of care for patients and relatives; the second is building up a united team; and the third is the development of each individual within the team, which includes the provision of physical, spiritual and emotional support, stimulus for learning and growth, leadership and job satisfaction. These three factors are obviously interdependent. Individual staff needs should rarely be given greater priority than the needs of patients or relatives, but equally, the needs of the team cannot always be neglected in favour of the maintenance of a high standard of care. It may sometimes be appropriate for the whole team to be put under more pressure, in order to support a particular individual. The keynote is clearly balance, and the maintenance of this balance is one of the vital functions of the team leader, who will usually be the ward sister or nursing officer.

ENVIRONMENT

A pleasant physical environment is very important for people involved in work as taxing as terminal care. Caring for someone in squalid housing conditions, particularly when incontinence or offensive lesions are a problem, can be a daunting prospect for the most committed nurse. Attempts at any major cleansing operation will almost certainly seem insensitive and inappropriate at such a time, and it is usually necessary to carry on regardless. Fortunately, the fast-growing complex of specialist units undertaking this type of work is largely composed of purpose-built, brand new buildings. Because of the emotive nature of the work, funds pour in and can be spent on the latest and best in hospital equipment, furniture and furnishings. Most units are single-storey buildings with easy access to surrounding gardens, overlooking trees, fields and golf courses. This can make a tremendous difference to staff confined in a fairly small area for eight or ten hours at a stretch, often in an atmosphere of great emotional tension and grief.

One cannot help but wonder how popular terminal care units would be to work in if they were sited on the fourth floor of an old city hospital, looking out onto brick walls and billowing chimneys, not to mention all the frustrations of out-dated, shoddy equipment, dingy paintwork, poor lighting and inadequate heating and ventilation. Many nurses are caring for dying patients on general wards in just those conditions. It is not surprising that some feel ambivalent towards the high ideals aspired to by many hospice nurses.

HEALTH

Each team member must be in good health, to be able to sustain the constant depth of emotional involvement and the strain of physically heavy nursing. Their need for a nourishing, balanced diet and adequate sleep and relaxation is paramount. Staff new to the work may well require guidance about holidays. They would be well advised to take short, frequent holidays at first, resisting the temptation of longer breaks taken less often. The latter so often results in sickness and absenteeism, due to the extreme exhaustion induced by working for the consequent long stretches without any respite.

When assessing the physical nursing needs of a group of terminally ill patients, they are seen to be comparable with those of thoracic surgery patients, the latter being the specialty usually cited as the most physically arduous sphere of nursing. In an average group of dying patients, approximately half will need a great deal of help with their personal care and a further quarter will be totally dependent. When one adds to this level of physical energy output all the stress factors inherent in terminal care, the need for staff who are physically and psychologically healthy becomes apparent. It is sometimes necessary to reject a candidate for a nursing post, whose personality and motivation seem ideally suited to the work, simply on grounds of physical frailty. This can be a painful decision, especially if remaining candidates appear second-rate by comparison, but one that is essential for the team as a whole. Other applicants who typically apply for work in terminal care, but who will need stealthily weeding out, are those whose motivation is their own unresolved grief (time since bereavement is no indication of the degree of resolution), those who are emotionally unstable and motivated by a desire to be part of a supportive community, primarily for their own needs, those with a morbid curiosity and those motivated by any form of evangelism. One is in no way seeking the perfect nurse; the very essence of a team is the way in which one person's strength compensates for another's weakness. However, there is a limit to the amount of support that staff can extend to one another in addition to the demands of the work.

JOB SATISFACTION

Every team member, whatever his or her qualifications, or lack of them, needs responsibility and autonomy in their work. One of the best ways of achieving this is total patient care, avoiding single task allocation as much as possible. In hospital, even simple things like cleaning rotas can be organised to give each person her own area of responsibility and pride, rather than anyone cleaning anything. The greater the challenge and the less oppressive the supervision, the more creative and conscientious will the care be.

At the end of forty-five minutes or an hour spent on the care of one patient, a wide variety of tasks will have been performed. This not only enriches the nurse's work, but the continuity of care will have enabled the patient to dictate both the order and the pace. To see a patient peacefully dozing off to sleep at the end of this time, and knowing that you alone are responsible for both his physical comfort and peace of mind, is one of the most satisfying moments of a nurse's day. In addition, this time span will be sufficient to facilitate the development and deepening of relationships, the aspect of nursing which makes it a caring profession rather than skilled manual work, and the aspect which provides the most job satisfaction of all.

Part of the role of the team leader is the provision of a stimulating, learning environment. Working with the dying is never boring; every patient presents a new set of problems and delights. To elicit the full potential of teaching material, however, it will be necessary to organise case conferences, persuade the staff to present case histories, and lead teaching rounds and report sessions. Formal teaching sessions, using films, slides, videos and cassettes, also have a useful role, as do discussion groups and seminars. Community staff and those caring for the dying on general wards will benefit greatly from either a visit or a longer period of experience in a specialist unit, whilst those working in the specialist units will benefit from visits to other relevant departments, such as radiotherapy and pain relief clinics. All hospital staff should be encouraged to experience community work as often as they can, to prevent the development of institutionalised attitudes. Every encouragement should also be given to those interested in undertaking any further training, and when possible funds should be allocated for staff to attend conferences and courses. Funds will also be needed for the provision of a comprehensive library and subscriptions for relevant magazines.

The most important teaching of all takes place at the bedside, however, not only in clinical demonstrations, but in the example set by more experienced colleagues of high quality communication with patients and relatives. It is salutary to remember that teaching by example is going on every moment of a working day.

RECOGNITION OF THE INDIVIDUAL

Every team member has a need for, and a right to, individual recognition. This can take many different forms. Time needs to be taken, particularly by the team leader, to get to know each person well, to know and enquire about their families and friends, to discover and hear about their interests and activities. This need never be considered as time-wasting, for how can staff be expected to treat patients as individuals, if they are simply numbers on the establishment list themselves?

The importance placed on family commitments, social events, evening classes, and the hundreds of other activities which fill the off-duty lives of each team member is made patently obvious by the amount of trouble and consideration given to the arrangement of duty rotas. All nurses are aware of the need for adequate ward coverage at all times, and most will willingly stand in for sick colleagues or help out at peak holiday periods, if they see that their own requests for special time off are being considered carefully and never refused unnecessarily.

The need for individual recognition may also be expressed in the team's desire to meet together from time to time in a social setting. This can take various forms: the traditional work Christmas party, a summer barbecue or barn dance, outings, meals in either restaurants or an individual's home, and social gatherings to mark the departure of a member of the team. Getting to know each other in this way, outside the work setting, can help to remove the barriers which can develop between those of different professions and status. This increased sense of equality and ease with one another enables the deepening of friendships, and the rounding off of relationships into richer, fuller and more normal shapes. If the preparation necessary for these events is delegated as widely as possible, the maximum number of people will benefit from the resulting sense of involvement. It may be a useful vehicle for integrating new or isolated members into the team.

Systems of hierarchy in nursing are unavoidable, since certain qualifications are necessary before various duties can be undertaken, and it is essential to delegate different levels of responsibility accordingly. But status has little meaning to dying patients; the nurse who is most important to them is the one with whom they develop the closest relationship, and this is just as likely to be the nursing auxiliary as the ward sister. If the emphasis on status is played down as far as possible, people are far more likely to feel valued for who they are, and for the unique contribution they make as human beings to the patients and their relatives, rather than for their qualifications or title.

Every individual needs constant reassurance, however competent and confident they may appear. Frequent validation of every member's performance is another vital task of the team leader. However, she too needs reassurance from the rest of the team to retain her own confidence and zest, rather than the all too common distancing and 'scapegoating' of those in a leadership role.

People need to know that it was noticed how sensitively they handled a particularly fraught family, how clearly they wrote up their patient's history, how conscientiously they cleaned and tidied up the sluice, or how scrupulously they carried out an aseptic technique. This is not only supportive to the individual, but is an investment for the future. With adequate praise and encouragement, standards of work will be maintained at a constantly high level. Time spent on validation of tasks performed well usually pays far greater dividends than time spent on negative criticism of faulty work.

A great deal of a nurse's individuality gets stamped on by the dogmatic approach of many training schools and by the need to conform to standard procedures and routines. In addition to this, because of the extreme 'busyness' of many wards and the lack of emphasis placed on teaching about human behaviour and relationships, nurses have a tendency to develop a set repertoire and manner, minimising the effort required to relate to patients. Unfortunately, the patients may find these as meaningless as the nurse who employs them.

Although the individuality of patients may be valued and respected in units specialising in the care of the dying, any display of behaviour in the staff which does not conform to the accepted prototype may well be rejected by the rest of the team, in a manner just as reactionary as that found in less enlightened wards. There is sometimes a remarkable lack of value placed on the individuality and slight eccentricities of colleagues, through a mistaken concern for the patient's well-being. Patients are almost invariably attracted to the more mischievous and irreverent members of staff. In order to overcome these pressures to conform, positive steps need taking to encourage individuality by constant appreciation of the whole nurse. The concept of caring for the whole patient may now seem quite acceptable, but the concept of a whole nurse may take rather longer to achieve respectability.

EMOTIONAL SUPPORT

THE COST OF CARING

Those who care for the dying have a great need themselves for emotional support. Each individual nurse will determine her own level of involvement, and this will vary widely. However, hospice staff are encouraged by the example of others to develop deep emotional bonds with patients and their families. Similar bonds are also likely to occur in the community, where only one or two nurses are caring for someone in the intimacy of their own home. But in the general hospitals, this depth of involvement is often disapproved of and considered to be unprofessional.

The value to the patient of close, trusting relationships has been demonstrated repeatedly, and it is essential that this should become more widely acknowledged and accepted by nurse managers. Only then will they begin to look at the emotional needs of nurses created by these relationships and seek ways of meeting them.

On the whole, the times of greatest suffering for patients are when they are coming to terms with the imminence of death, when they deteriorate physically and lose their independence, and when pain or other symptoms are unrelieved. Consequently, these are the times when the nurse who is closely involved is likely to suffer the most too, and death itself may be a blessed relief. Nevertheless, however welcome the death may be, the nurse is still bereaved in just the same way as she would be following the death of anyone else with whom she has had a close relationship. Many of the emotions described in the previous chapter will be aroused. Guilt is a frequent component of a nurse's bereavement; guilt at not having been more tolerant or not having done more for the patient. Anger is also common; anger with God or anger with the doctors who failed to effect a cure. There is often a great deal of difficulty in relating to a new patient who has been admitted into the bed previously occupied by someone who has recently died.

The depth of involvement with each individual patient will obviously determine the nature of the bereavement, as will the length of time that the relationship has existed. Staff working with long-stay patients, such as the young disabled, the chronic sick, geriatrics, or the mentally subnormal, are almost certain to grieve more at a patient's death than a nurse in a coronary care unit. Understanding and recognition of this grief, acceptance of its normality, and support to work through it are essential in every situation where nurses are caring for patients who may die. Those working in terminal care units tend to develop extremely close relationships with the patients in a very short period of time, therefore their need for emotional support is often as great as those caring for longer-stay patients.

Nurses who take on a counselling role learn to empathise with patients and relatives at a very deep level. Consequently, they 'take on board' a great deal of the client's pain and suffering. It is essential for these feelings to be worked through and vented regularly.

Of course, people who are dying are not always 'nice'. They are just as likely to be aggressive, hypercritical, self-pitying or demanding as anyone else, and it is not at all unusual for them to displace their anger about dying onto those who are caring for them. It is one thing to be able to understand intellectually why a patient is being so unpleasant, but it is quite another to refrain from acting on hurt feelings, either by retaliating or by withdrawing from the relationship. The sensitive support of colleagues is essential.

When nurses are constantly surrounded by people who are dying, they are at risk of becoming irrationally anxious about their own health. Every symptom can be diagnosed as a fatal disease, and some nurses have recurrent nightmares about dying. Embarrassment and fear of being ridiculed often cause these matters to be concealed, or else to be raised in a jocular manner, but the fears may be deep, and a caring, thoughtful response is called for. Encouragement to seek medical advice and a thorough physical examination may be more effective than countless counselling sessions.

MEETING THE NEEDS

Having looked at the kind of emotional cost involved in nursing people who are dying, it is important to look at some of the practical frameworks which can be used in the provision of emotional support.

A stable, permanent team, rather than one whose members are periodically re-allocated to other wards and departments, is essential. This is especially true of work in the community, where supportive contact with colleagues is much less easily available. Given this degree of permanence, deep relationships can form between members and the best form of emotional support can be given and received, namely friendship.

When one nursing shift hands over to another, a fairly lengthy and detailed report session can combine support with a useful exchange of important information. Those members of staff who have been providing the care and support for the patients have an opportunity to share their experiences with the newly arrived staff and to express any relevant thoughts or feelings. Although the report session may be led by the senior nurse on duty, every member of the team should be encouraged to make their own contribution.

A liaison psychiatrist or medical social worker, slightly removed from the ward team, can be a great asset. They may well be able to perceive relationship problems with patients far more objectively than those submerged in the work. By using group sessions, difficult or strange behaviour can be explored and understood more clearly. The member of staff who is experiencing the difficulty can often be helped by bringing any negative feelings about the patient out into the open. They may previously have been experiencing a considerable amount of guilt. It may also be possible to uncover the reason for their particular difficulty with a specific patient. Increased understanding of both her own and the patient's feelings frequently results in more tolerant and effective care.

Ideally, all nurses should have regular appraisal sessions with the senior nurse in their team. This can be an excellent time for unearthing worries and difficulties. When a group of nurses is continually giving of itself to the extent advocated in this book, they will need and deserve leaders who are prepared to treat these sessions as a high priority. To make appraisal sessions an effective framework for providing support, whilst remaining practicable for the busy team leader, three months will probably be about the right interval of time to allow between them. Every nurse needs to know that she will be given time immediately if she becomes distressed or overwhelmed by her work. She must also know that she can count on genuine care and concern, with no fear of mockery, criticism or a lack of sensitivity and understanding. In many wards and hospices, the senior nurses, the chaplain, the social worker and, where there is one, the psychiatrist, will all make themselves available to individual nurses in need of this type of support. It will usually take the form of counselling sessions.

There is a great need for respect and trust between all the different disciplines of staff, but perhaps especially between doctors and nurses. Decisions, whenever possible, should be made jointly, but when of necessity they are made alone, they should be made in complete confidence that they will be supported and upheld. One such decision that is very much involved with the emotional thermometer of the team is the allocation of beds. After a particularly traumatic few days with sudden, frequent or young deaths, when staff numbers are low due to sickness or holidays, the morale of the whole staff can reach rock bottom. A sensitive doctor, responsible for arranging admissions, will tread gently in accepting new patients if other hospital beds are available. It is of little value admitting patients, however needy, if the staff are too drained emotionally to offer them the care that they require. Similarly, in the community, the time may come when the small team of nursing staff involved are physically and emotionally incapable of continuing to care for a dying patient at home. The support and understanding of the general practitioner is vital in such an event.

The need for emotional support will not always be met within the working environment. Many nurses will find their own means of venting the painful feelings which have been stored up. Some will be able to work through them by sharing them with a close friend or their family. Others will find that this puts too great a strain on their relationships, since the need will be a constant one, so they look elsewhere for help. Some will be able to use prayer and the support of a priest. Others will seek the help of a professional counsellor or therapist.

Nurses, along with others involved in 'caring professions', whose functioning at work needs to be on a deeper emotional level than in most other fields, are becoming increasingly aware of their need for emotional as well as physical refreshment. This would seem to be one of the main reasons why yoga, relaxation techniques, meditation and some of the recently developed forms of self-help therapy are gaining popularity so fast, although they are not, of course, in any way confined to the 'caring professions'. A hearty choir practice, a game of tennis or a long country walk will also reduce tension and the physical symptoms it produces, but their results are not as impressive as those produced by the techniques specifically designed to release stress.

MAINTAINING THE BALANCE

There is a vital balance which everyone caring for those who are suffering in any way must be able to maintain. Although they must have the ability to be open enough to empathise, and consequently to get hurt by their involvement, they must also be strong enough to avoid being damaged. The competent team leader will be as aware of each individual's emotional condition as she possibly can. Although signs of stress will usually indicate the need for a break or for additional help, aimed at enabling the individual to continue in the same field of work, support to move on to a different type of work may be more appropriate if these signs should become severe or prolonged, indicating that a more damaging effect is occurring. The most common warning lights are deterioration in family and social relationships, withdrawal from outside activities as these begin to seem inappropriate when surrounded by death and dying, an over-intense involvement with patients that is allowed to encroach into a great deal of the person's off-duty hours, and a very high level of persistent fatigue.

Some nurses simply refuse to recognise their own emotional needs, thus failing to obtain any means of support outside the working environment and rejecting any offer of help within it. If they then open themselves to the pain and suffering of their patients, they may eventually reach saturation point. When this occurs they may try to continue working at the same depth and with the same openness, in which case they are likely to become ill, either physically or emotionally. Alternatively and quite unconsciously they may employ defence mechanisms to prevent the arousal of painful feelings. Although they may appear to be as caring as they ever were, the patients will sense the barrier and may find themselves unable to share their feelings at anything like the previous depth. Experienced members of the team may be aware of what is happening, but it is not always possible to persuade people to accept the help which they clearly need.

One of the greatest emotional needs, but probably one least thought about in terminal care, is the need for humour. It rarely offends either patients or relatives to see the staff enjoying a good laugh, especially if they are included. Of course it is necessary to use discretion in the presence of grieving families or confused patients, who may think themselves the focus of the humour, but a hushed, humourless atmosphere can be very oppressive for patients, families and staff. There are few better ways of relieving tension and strain than laughter.

COUNSELLING

The value of counselling, as one of the tools that can be used in the care of dying patients and those who are close to them, has been alluded to in every chapter of this book. However, it also has an important role to play in the care of the nurse.

The nursing team's need for counselling falls into three major categories. Firstly, support in coping with the emotional stress implicit in their daily work; secondly, support in coping with personal matters; and thirdly, a quite different mode of counselling necessitated by the more formal interview situations, as in appointment of staff, termination of employment and, when necessary, disciplining staff.

The skills required for the latter type of counselling are likely to be developed on courses in management. Procedural guidelines are usually laid down by the personnel department of the employing authority. Perhaps the one formal counselling situation which requires elaboration here is the disciplinary procedure, as this strikes a rather incongruous note after the previous accounts of emotional support. This can be one of the leader's most difficult undertakings in the context of a caring team. However, if there is any evidence of misconduct or incompetence amongst the staff, the team leader must have the confidence and ability to confront and, if necessary, reprimand them. This should be undertaken in privacy and within strict bounds of confidentiality. Even criticism can be expressed caringly, explanations for misconduct being sought and listened to attentively. When working alongside the staff member concerned, following a disciplinary counselling session, the close nature of the nursing team may cause embarrassment on both sides. It is the responsibility of the counsellor to act in a relaxed way in her dealings with the person concerned, making it quite clear that no ill-feeling is being harboured and that their previous good relationship is unaffected.

A confident and caring disciplinary session will usually need no repetition, but validation of improved efforts is essential. Failure to produce any improvement will probably necessitate referral to more senior staff and the implementation for more formal disciplinary action. The other side of this coin is, of course, the use of the grievance procedures available to all staff. However great the provocation, it is important that those in more senior positions avoid any harrassing behaviour which might constitute 'constructive dismissal'. This occurs when an individual resigns from her job because the atmosphere or conditions make it no longer possible for her to continue. Sadly, this type of behaviour is now not uncommon, since the tightening of employment legislation has made the dismissal of staff more difficult.

The less formal, therapeutic form of counselling, already described in Chapter 4, can be used to meet many of the emotional needs described in the previous section.

The line between counselling and supportive sharing in a work group is sometimes difficult to draw, hence the importance of being explicit about which information is to be treated as confidential and which is not. It can be devastating to discover that a confidence has been betrayed, however innocently or unwittingly it was done.

Counselling staff with major or protracted personal problems can be very time-consuming, and is not always an appropriate use of the team leader's time. It is important to know one's own limitations in this field and also to be aware of the existence of local counselling services to which staff may need to be referred.

SPIRITUAL AND ETHICAL MATTERS

The spiritual needs of a nursing team should never be overlooked. Faith can be so easily shaken by the awareness of so much suffering, and many spiritual questions may be provoked by the constant presence of death and dying.

Questions of a moral or ethical nature will arise with predictable regularity. These questions may be related to a specific patient and his family, or they may be those which are of general concern in terminal care. They may include the question of confidentiality. When, for example, should information imparted to a member of staff go no further than that one person, and when is it right to share this information with the rest of the team, enabling more informed and thus more effective care to be given? They may include questions about the right of patients to obtain euthanasia, or the use of drugs to suppress consciousness when physical or mental pain is not amenable to other forms of treatment. They may include questions about the morality of telling a patient that he is going to die soon, or the morality of withholding life-prolonging treatments.

There should be a time when these matters can be discussed freely by both believing and non-believing members of the team together. Team members have a great need to share thoughts and feelings about this type of question, in the knowledge that they will be listened to carefully and respected. Any team is likely to contain conflicting ideas, and general agreement may not be reached. Discussion should not be dominated by a single approach, neither the one which represents the majority view, nor that of the senior members, whether this be Christian, agnostic or something else.

For many members of the caring team, their work is part of their Christian commitment. For these people, prayer groups can be fundamental to their needs. Here they may communally offer up their work to God and pray for his support and guidance. Sensitivity towards the feelings of non-believing colleagues is necessary, however, to prevent such meetings from appearing elitist or exclusive, particularly when the more senior members of staff are involved. Similarly, sensitivity and respect for the beliefs and spiritual needs of their colleagues should be forthcoming from the non-believers in the team. Those who hold a faith other than Christianity will also need support. Since they are likely to be few and far between, it would be quite possible for all members of the team to be fairly well informed about the beliefs of their colleagues, thus preventing feelings of isolation.

The hospital chaplain may play an important role in facilitating both the discussion group and the prayer meeting. No two teams will have the same needs, and the chaplain who is closely involved may be the most suitable person to decide how best to meet the particular needs of the team. He may also be of great value in the support of individual members of staff who are under particular strain, or whose faith is undergoing changes because of their frequent contact with death and mourning. Unlike the counselling support provided by other colleagues, pastoral counselling fosters not only the relationship between the minister and the client, but also between the client and God. It is as dependent upon prayer as it is upon an expertise in counselling. Those caring for the dying will need help to find, either from within themselves or from their God, the strength which they require to sustain themselves.

LEADERSHIP

In this description of the needs of the nursing team, the role of the team leader in meeting these needs has been mentioned repeatedly. Most often this role will be filled by the ward sister. In the community nursing service and in some hospices it may be the nursing officer or matron who is best able to meet these needs. Where groups of nurses of a similar status are working closely together with their immediate superior based some distance away, such as staff nurses on night duty or sisters working on the district, a natural leader will very often emerge within the group. Occasionally the general practitioner or the hospital or hospice consultant will take on a leadership role. However, this leadership is generally confined to medical concerns, with nursing and personal leadership being sought elsewhere.

Leadership carries many unpleasant connotations of hierarchy systems, authoritarianism and strict discipline. This is quite obviously not what is needed from the leaders of a caring team, but they do fulfil a very important function. Their most important role is to encourage growth and the development of autonomy and self-discipline, whilst ensuring that the highest possible standard of patient care is maintained. To achieve both these ends, the leader will be required not only to offer the quality of support already described, but also to set an example of excellence in her own work. In a relaxed, informal atmosphere, where everyone is treated with mutual respect, the leader's own high standards, though in no way forced upon the other team members, will invariably motivate them to emulation.

A team leader should never confine herself to a rigid, limited number of tasks. She should regularly undertake every type of work that is required of the other members, thus demonstrating both her respect for the work and the standard she expects of others. Just as no task should be beneath her dignity, similarly no task should be considered too important to delegate. It is usually a lack of confidence and competence which makes delegation difficult.

To list the personal qualities required for leadership is increasingly thought to be inappropriate and unhelpful. Three which do warrant mentioning, however, are sensitivity, integrity and self-awareness. All three are equally important, but self-awareness may be the hardest to achieve. By the very nature of their role, leaders are unlikely to get feedback on their own performance with the same frankness that the other members of the team will receive it from their peers (although this can be possible in a non-authoritarian group). Responsibility will therefore rest heavily on the leader for monitoring her own interactions with the team and with the individuals in it.

Because of the extra pressure and responsibility on those in leadership roles, it is particularly important that they should feel appreciated, at least as much as they are criticised.

REFERENCE

Adair, John, *Action Centred Leadership*. McGraw-Hill, 1973.

RECOMMENDED FURTHER READING

DEATH AND DYING

Feifel, Herman, *New Meanings of Death*. McGraw-Hill, 1959.
Hinton, John, *Dying*. Pelican, 1967.
Huntingdon and Metcalf, *Celebrations of Death*. Cambridge University Press, 1979.
Kübler-Ross, Elizabeth, *On Death and Dying*. Tavistock, 1973.
Mansell Patterson, E., *The Experience of Dying*. McGraw-Hill, 1959.
Toynbee, A. et al., *Man's Concern with Death*. Hodder and Stoughton, 1968.

TERMINAL CARE

Ainsworth-Smith, I. and Speck, P., *Letting Go*. SPCK, 1982.
Downie, P. A., *Cancer Rehabilitation*. Faber, 1976.
Lamerton, Richard, *Care of the Dying*. Penguin, 1980.
Poss, Sylvia, *Towards Death With Dignity*. Allen and Unwin, 1981.
Saunders, C. (ed.), *The Management of Terminal Disease*. Edward Arnold, 1978.
Saunders, C. M., Summers, Dorothy H. and Teller, Neville, (co-editors), *Hospice - The Living Idea*. Edward Arnold, 1981.
Stoddard, Sandol, *The Hospice Movement*. Jonathan Cape, 1978.
Terminal Care, A Nursing Times Reprint. Macmillan Journals, 1971.

DYING CHILDREN

Bluebond-Langner, Myra, *The Private Worlds of Dying Children*. Princeton University Press, 1978.
Burton, L., *Care of the Child Facing Death*. Routledge and Kegan Paul, 1974.
Gyulay, Jo-Eileen, *The Dying Child*. McGraw-Hill, 1978.

Bond, M. R., *Pain - Its Nature, Analysis and Treatment*. Churchill-Livingstone, 1979.
Eldersbee, M., *Taught by Pain*. Falcon, 1970.
Malzack, Ronald, *The Puzzle of Pain*. Penguin, 1973.
McCaffery, Margaret, *Nursing Management of the Patient with Pain*. Lippincott, 1972.

CANCER

Burn, Ian and Meyrick, Roger (co-editors), *Understanding Cancer - A Guide for the Caring Professionals*. D.H.S.S., H.M.S.O., 1977.
Capra, L. G., *Care of the Cancer Patient*. Heinemann, 1972.
Scott, Bodley, *Cancer - The Facts*. Oxford University Press, 1979.
Tiffany, Robert, *Oncology for Nurses and Health Care Professionals*, Parts 1 and 2. Allen and Unwin, 1978.

BEREAVEMENT

Bowlby, John, *Loss, Sadness and Depression* (Volume 3 of *Attachment and Loss*). Hogarth Press, 1980.
Furman, E., *A Child's Parent Dies*. Yale, 1974.
Murray Parkes, C., *Bereavement*. Pelican, 1975.
Pincus, Lily, *Life and Death*. Abacus, 1976.
Smith, Kathleen, *Help for the Bereaved*. Duckworth, 1978.

PERSONAL ACCOUNTS OF DYING AND BEREAVEMENT

De Beauvoir, S., *A Very Easy Death*. Penguin, 1964.
Evans, J., *Living with a Man who is Dying*. Blond, 1971.
Hill, Susan, *In the Springtime of the Year*. Penguin, 1974.
Lewis, C. S., *A Grief Observed*. Faber and Faber, 1961.
Paton, Alan, *Kontakion for You Departed*. Jonathan Cape, 1969.
Stevans, S., *Death Comes Home*. Mowbray, 1972.
Torrie, Margaret, *Begin Again, Book for Women Alone*. Dent, 1970.
Zorza, Rosemary and Victor, *A Way to Die: Living to the End*. Andre Deutsch, 1980.

COMMUNICATION AND COUNSELLING

McIntosh, T., *Communication and Awareness in a Cancer Ward*. Croom-Helm, 1977.
Nurse, Gaynor, *Counselling and the Nurse*. HM & M, 1980.
Proctor, Brigid, *Counselling Shop*. Andre Deutsch, 1978.
Venables, Ethel, *Counselling*. National Marriage Guidance Council, 1971.
Storr, Anthony, *The Art of Psychotherapy*. Secker and Warburg/Heinemann, 1979.
Tschudin, Verena, *Counselling Skills for Nurses*. Baillière Tindall, 1982.

GENERAL INTEREST

Illich, Ivan, *Limits to Medicine*. Pelican, 1976.
Moody, Raymond, *Life After Life*. Corgi, 1975.
Stockwell, F., *The Unpopular Patient*. Royal College of Nursing, 1972.
Solzhenitsyn, A., *Cancer Ward*. Bodley Head, 1968.
Wilson, Michael, *Health is for People*. Darton, Longman and Todd, 1975.
Winefield, H. R. and Peay, M. Y., *Behavioural Science in Medicine*. Allen and Unwin/Beaconsfield, 1980.

QUESTIONS FOR STUDY AND REFLECTION

1) Is death a taboo subject, and if so, what effect does it have on our society?

2) How do cultural and religious differences affect attitudes towards death?

3) Why did the hospice movement come into being? What contribution has it made and in which direction should it be developing?

4) Why is individualised care so hard to achieve in a hospital ward, and how can the difficulties be overcome?

5) What are the underlying principles upon which high standards of care for the dying depend?

6) Good communication between the dying and those caring for them is essential. What are the factors which facilitate and enhance it?

7) In order to come to terms with the knowledge that death is imminent, a major psychological adjustment is necessary. How can a nurse assist this process?

8) What is pain?

9) What are the main principles to be considered when prescribing analgesics for the terminally ill?

10) 'There is nothing more that we can do.' This statement is made, not uncommonly, when curative treatment has failed, but why should it always be challenged?

11) Why is it that providing physical nursing care for the dying is so rewarding?

12) 'Thou shalt not kill but needst not strive officiously to keep alive.' (From the Hippocratic oath.) If this guidance was adhered to more often, how would the euthanasia debate be affected?

13) Is it ever possible for the grief of a bereavement to be resolved, and what would such a resolution entail?

14) 'Do you specialise in any particular field of nursing?' 'Yes, the care of the dying.' 'Oh, how depressing.' This is rarely true, but why not?

Index